K. Jean Peterson, DSW
Editor

Health Care for Lesbians and Gay Men: Confronting Homophobia and Heterosexism

*Pre-publication
REVIEWS,
COMMENTARIES,
EVALUATIONS . . .*

" . . . [T]his book is an eye-opener. Documented with both scholarly literature and real-life examples, the book leaves no doubt that much of our current health care delivery system is fraught with bias and homophobia.

This book should be read by all of us in social work, regardless of our professed area of interest or field of service."

Alice A. Lieberman, PhD, LMSW
Associate Professor and Chair, BSW Program, University of Kansas

D1056561

Health Care for Lesbians and Gay Men: Confronting Homophobia and Heterosexism

Health Care for Lesbians and Gay Men: Confronting Homophobia and Heterosexism

K. Jean Peterson, DSW
Editor

Health Care for Lesbians and Gay Men: Confronting Homophobia and Heterosexism, edited by K. Jean Peterson, was simultaneously issued by The Haworth Press, Inc., under the same title, as a special issue of *Journal of Gay & Lesbian Social Services,* Volume 5, Number 1 1996, James J. Kelly, Editor.

Harrington Park Press
An Imprint of
The Haworth Press, Inc.
New York • London

1-56023-079-7

Published by

Harrington Park Press, 10 Alice Street, Binghamton, NY 13904-1580 USA

Harrington Park Press is an imprint of The Haworth Press, Inc.,10 Alice Street, Binghamton, NY 13904-1580 USA.

Health Care for Lesbians and Gay Men: Confronting Homophobia and Heterosexism has also been published as *Journal of Gay & Lesbian Social Services*, Volume 5, Number 1 1996.

Library of Congress Cataloging-in-Publication Data

Health care for lesbians and gay men: confronting homophobia and heterosexism/ K. Jean Peterson, editor.
     p. cm.
     "Also published as Journal of gay & lesbian social services, volume 5, number 1, 1996" –T.p. verso.
     Includes bibliographical references and index.
     ISBN 1-56024-772-X (THP : alk. paper). – ISBN 1-56023-079-7 (HPP: alk. paper)
     1. Gays–Medical care. 2. Gays-Health and hygiene. 3. Heterosexism. 4. Homophobia I. Peterson, K. Jean. II. Journal of gay & lesbian social services.
RA564.9.H65H43 1996
362.1'08'664–dc20
                             95-23147
                               CIP

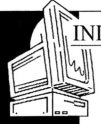

INDEXING & ABSTRACTING

Contributions to this publication are selectively indexed or abstracted in print, electronic, online, or CD-ROM version(s) of the reference tools and information services listed below. This list is current as of the copyright date of this publication. See the end of this section for additional notes.

- *AIDS Newsletter c/o CAB International/CAB ACCESS . . . available in print, diskettes updated weekly, and on INTERNET. Providing full bibliographic listings, author affiliation, augmented keyword searching,* CAB International, P.O. Box 100, Wallingford Oxon OX10 8DE, United Kingdom

- *Cambridge Scientific Abstracts, Risk Abstracts,* Environmental Routenet (accessed via INTERNET), 7200 Wisconsin Avenue #601, Bethesda, MD 20814

- *caredata CD: the social and community care database,* National Institute for Social Work, 5 Tavistock Place, London WC1H 9SS, England

- *CNPIEC Reference Guide: Chinese National Directory of Foreign Periodicals,* P.O. Box 88, Beijing, People's Republic of China

- *Digest of Neurology and Psychiatry,* The Institute of Living, 400 Washington Street, Hartford, CT 06106

- *ERIC Clearinghouse on Urban Education (ERIC/CUE),* Teachers College, Columbia University, Box 40, New York, NY 10027

- *Family Life Educator "Abstracts Section,"* ETR Associates, P.O. Box 1830, Santa Cruz, CA 95061-1830

- *Family Studies Database (online and CD/ROM)* Peters Technology Transfer, 306 East Baltimore Pike, 2nd Floor, Media, PA 19063

- *HOMODOK/"Relevant" Bibliographic database, Documentation Centre for Gay & Lesbian Studies, University of Amsterdam (selective printed abstracts in "Homologie" and bibliographic computer databases covering cultural, historical, social and political aspects of gay and lesbian topics)* % HOMODOK-ILGA Archive, O.Z. Achterburgwal 185, NL-1012 DK Amsterdam, The Netherlands

(continued)

- *IBZ International Bibliography of Periodical Literature,* Zeller Verlag GmbH & Co., P.O.B. 1949, d-49009, Osnabruck, Germany

- *Index to Periodical Articles Related to Law,* University of Texas, 727 East 26th Street, Austin, TX 78705

- *INTERNET ACCESS (& additional networks) Bulletin Board for Libraries ("BUBL"), coverage of information resources on INTERNET, JANET, and other networks.*
  - JANET X.29: UK.AC.BATH.BUBL or 00006012101300
  - TELNET: BUBL.BATH.AC.UK or 138.38.32.45 login 'bubl'
  - Gopher: BUBL.BATH.AC.UK (138.32.32.45). Port 7070
  - World Wide Web: http: / / www.bubl.bath.ac.uk./BUBL/ home.html
  - NISSWAIS: telnetniss.ac.uk (for the NISS gateway)

  The Andersonian Library, Curran Building, 101 St. James Road, Glasgow G4 ONS, Scotland

- *Mental Health Abstracts (online through DIALOG),* IFI/Plenum Data Company, 3202 Kirkwood Highway, Wilmington, DE 19808

- *Referativnyi Zhurnal (Abstracts Journal of the Institute of Scientific Information of the Republic of Russia),* The Institute of Scientific Information, Baltijskaja ul., 14, Moscow A-219, Republic of Russia

- *Social Work Abstracts,* National Association of Social Workers, 750 First Street NW, 8th Floor, Washington, DC 20002

- *Sociological Abstracts (SA),* Sociological Abstracts, Inc., P.O. Box 22206, San Diego, CA 92192-0206

- *Studies on Women Abstracts,* Carfax Publishing Company, P.O. Box 25, Abingdon, Oxfordshire OX14 3UE, United Kingdom

- *Violence and Abuse Abstracts: A Review of Current Literature on Interpersonal Violence (VAA),* Sage Publications, Inc., 2455 Teller Road, Newbury Park, CA 91320

(continued)

SPECIAL BIBLIOGRAPHIC NOTES

related to special journal issues (separates)
and indexing/abstracting

☐ indexing/abstracting services in this list will also cover material in any "separate" that is co-published simultaneously with Haworth's special thematic journal issue or DocuSerial. Indexing/abstracting usually covers material at the article/chapter level.

☐ monographic co-editions are intended for either non-subscribers or libraries which intend to purchase a second copy for their circulating collections.

☐ monographic co-editions are reported to all jobbers/wholesalers/approval plans. The source journal is listed as the "series" to assist the prevention of duplicate purchasing in the same manner utilized for books-in-series.

☐ to facilitate user/access services all indexing/abstracting services are encouraged to utilize the co-indexing entry note indicated at the bottom of the first page of each article/chapter/contribution.

☐ this is intended to assist a library user of any reference tool (whether print, electronic, online, or CD-ROM) to locate the monographic version if the library has purchased this version but not a subscription to the source journal.

☐ individual articles/chapters in any Haworth publication are also available through the Haworth Document Delivery Services (HDDS).

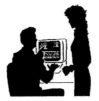

CONTENTS

ABOUT THE EDITOR

K. Jean Peterson, DSW, is Associate Professor at the University of Kansas School of Social Welfare in Lawrence, Kansas. Her scholarly interests have long been in the area of social work practice in health care, with a recent emphasis on social work practice with persons with HIV/AIDS. Dr. Peterson is a consulting editor of *Social Work, Smith College Studies in Social Work,* and *Journal of Gay & Lesbian Social Services.* She is also a long time member of the Council on Social Work Education, the National Association of Social Workers, and a past member of the Society of Hospital Social Work Directors.

Foreword

RATIONING BY SILENCE AND IGNORANCE

Creating a system of universal coverage became one of the key issues in the recent debate about American health care reform. As a profession, social work strongly supports the principle of universal access and coverage. Unfortunately, discrimination against certain groups in the American system leads to the unintended (or intended) consequence of excluding members of these groups from coverage as well as promoting the system's failure to address their unique needs.

For such oppressed groups, what emerges is a rationing of sorts. Many nations ration services and coverage in their health care systems. Although rationing is usually thought of as a reasoned, formal, and agreed upon approach to limit coverage to certain people and/or not develop selected health care services, a powerful informal means of rationing and restriction exists within American health care. While the American debate on rationing still focuses on whether or not to ration, it ignores the reality that the American system rations services and coverage according to factors such as geography, income, ethnicity, and/or social status.

Using discriminatory attitudes and practices to ration access to and creation of services within health care has had an especially negative impact on the lives and health of lesbian and gay people. The delivery of health care to lesbian and gay Americans is severely

---

Dean Pierce, PhD, is Director, Department of Social Work, University of Nevada-Reno, BB 525, Reno, NV 89557-0068.

[Haworth co-indexing entry note]: "Foreword." Pierce, Dean. Co-published simultaneously in *Journal of Gay & Lesbian Social Services* (The Haworth Press, Inc.) Vol. 5, No. 1, 1996, pp. xv-xvii; and: *Health Care for Lesbians and Gay Men: Confronting Homophobia and Heterosexism* (ed: K. Jean Peterson) The Haworth Press, Inc., 1996, pp. xiii-xv; and: *Health Care for Lesbians and Gay Men: Confronting Homophobia and Heterosexism* (ed: K. Jean Peterson) Harrington Park Press, an imprint of The Haworth Press, Inc., 1996, pp. xiii-xv. Single or multiple copies of this article are available from The Haworth Document Delivery Service [1-800-342-9678, 9:00 a.m. - 5:00 p.m. (EST)].

rationed: individual access is limited and the unique needs of this population are inadequately addressed. For example, the response of our health care system at the beginning of the AIDS crisis clearly reflects our system's unstated policy of rationing services according to stigma and social worth.

Moreover, the pattern of rationing of health care to lesbian and gay people has not been addressed. Although health care reform is a powerful political topic, the ongoing debate on American health care, strengthened by the President's reform proposal, has been inaccurate, ignorant, or silent regarding issues of lesbian and gay health. Health care reform discussions have only minimally addressed the status and needs of lesbian and gay people in the system.

Central to this rationing is America's bigotry and fear regarding homosexuality and homosexual people. This fear and bigotry result in a chilling silence: homosexual people do not speak up when they are patients and the health care system itself remains unresponsive to the unique needs of lesbian and gay people.

The phenomenon of silence about lesbians and gays in American health care reflects the deep-seated heterosexism and homophobia of American culture and its social institutions. Heterosexism has silenced many lesbians and gays, preventing them from advocating for their unique needs when they are patients in the system. In addition, professional ignorance and fear regarding lesbian and gay health needs has reinforced this silence and further hampered effective and helpful reforms.

If a cross section of Americans, including social workers, were asked to talk about lesbian and gay people in the American health care system, it is quite likely that their comments would focus almost exclusively on gay men and AIDS. Much of their discussion would reflect their fear of homosexuality and AIDS, not their knowledge about AIDS. It is also likely that the current discussion of health care reform by America's political leaders and health care professionals would inadequately attend to the needs of lesbian and gay people.

UNIQUE NEEDS

The slow pace of the health care system in creating services to meet lesbian and gay health care needs has been exacerbated by the unwillingness or reluctance of policy makers and health care professionals to accept the idea that the needs of lesbian and gay people differ from those of heterosexuals. Armed with the belief that there are no differences, lesbians and gays receive less than adequate and effective services from professionals who base services and treatments on needs other than those of their lesbian and gay patients.

Lesbian and gay people share common health care needs with other citizens, yet also require the provision of care to cover their unique needs. As noted above, access is denied through the power and negativism of heterosexism. In addition, this attitude masks the unique needs of lesbian and gay people. For example, heterosexist attitudes and practices have dismissed the unique needs of lesbians regarding the high risk for breast cancer and they have been slow to recognize the place and uniqueness of lesbian and gay people in substance abuse programs. Similarly, insurance coverage does not extend to lesbian and gay couples.

Compounding this problem are the great differences between lesbians and gays as well as the differences among lesbians within their communities and among gays within theirs. Hence, just as health care needs are ignored or denied, the cultural context of lesbian and gay health care needs is seldom considered.

CONCLUSION

The articles in this collection go far toward addressing the uniqueness of lesbian and gay health care needs and add significantly to our knowledge of needed and existing programs and services. The solutions offered by the authors are substantive and sophisticated. They offer practical interventions; call for advocacy, social change, grassroots efforts, and alternative programs; and provide lessons about how to use existing procedures more effectively to meet the unique needs of lesbian and gay people. The authors cover information on making and protecting health care decisions and using legal approaches to secure and maintain patients' wishes regarding personal health care.

Dean Pierce, PhD

Preface:
Developing the Context:
The Impact of Homophobia
and Heterosexism on the Health Care
of Gay and Lesbian People

Homophobia and heterosexism are rampant throughout the health care industry. Blatant homophobia is manifested through the negative treatment of gay and lesbian youth and adults. Whether it be the dismissal by the physician of a gay man experiencing impotency (see Schwartz in this issue), or the refusal of a physician to complete the physical exam of a woman who discloses her lesbianism (Smith, Johnson, & Guenther, 1985), the impact on health care is clear. Lesbians and gay men receive inferior treatment from providers who are homophobic. In addition, because of these negative experiences with providers, lesbians seek health care less frequently (Robertson & Schachter, 1981), and most likely the same is true with gay men.

Heterosexism can have an equally deleterious effect on the health care received by gays and lesbians. The assumption of heterosexuality by providers results in inadequate information being available for diagnosis, and compromised treatment and aftercare.

K. Jean Peterson, DSW, is Associate Professor, School of Social Welfare, University of Kansas, Lawrence, KS 66045-2510.

[Haworth co-indexing entry note]: "Preface: Developing the Context: The Impact of Homophobia and Heterosexism on the Health Care of Gay and Lesbian People." Peterson, K. Jean. Co-published simultaneously in *Journal of Gay & Lesbian Social Services* (The Haworth Press, Inc.) Vol. 5, No. 1, 1996, pp. xix-xxii; and: *Health Care for Lesbians and Gay Men: Confronting Homophobia and Heterosexism* (ed: K. Jean Peterson) The Haworth Press, Inc., 1996, pp. xvii-xx; and: *Health Care for Lesbians and Gay Men: Confronting Homophobia and Heterosexism* (ed: K. Jean Peterson) Harrington Park Press, an imprint of The Haworth Press, Inc., 1996, pp. xvii-xx. Single or multiple copies of this article are available from The Haworth Document Delivery Service [1-800-342-9678, 9:00 a.m. - 5:00 p.m. (EST)].

xvii

The impact of homophobia and heterosexism in health care is evident across the life span of gay and lesbian people. In this volume, Gochros and Bidwell document the effect on gay and lesbian youth, who may manifest their struggles with sexual identity through alcohol and drug abuse, as well as a higher incidence of suicide. Without the knowledge of the youths' sexual orientation and struggles, health care providers risk misdiagnosis and inadequate treatment planning. In addition, gay and lesbian youth are at higher risk for being the victims of violent acts due to pervasive societal homophobia. Along with discussing the plight of gay and lesbian youth, Gochros and Bidwell discuss the development of comprehensive programs which address the physical, psychological, social and spiritual needs of these youth.

Schwartz looks more directly at the impact of homophobia and heterosexism on gay men within the health care system and the resulting impact on care. The AIDS crisis has resulted in these issues being acted out more blatantly than in the past, with physicians and nurses acknowledging "more negative, even overtly hostile, feelings towards homosexuals than they had before the emergence of the AIDS epidemic" (Douglas, Kalman, & Kalman, 1985, p. 1311). Schwartz, proposing solutions, calls upon gay men to inform local, state and national organizations about unethical medical practices and to actively work on their own internalized homophobia to overcome a passive stance to inadequate care.

Peterson and Bricker-Jenkins, along with Levy, look at the impact of homophobia and heterosexism on lesbians. In addition to discussing the health care-seeking behaviors of lesbians, and the barriers lesbians encounter in obtaining health care, Peterson and Bricker-Jenkins look specifically at how these attitudes and beliefs affect both the diagnosis and care of lesbians with breast cancer. Levy, discussing reproductive issues for lesbians, looks at not only the impact of homophobia and heterosexism on prenatal and postpartum care, but also the effect on the definition of family.

The effect of heterosexism and homophobia on both the assessment and treatment of alcohol and drug abuse is discussed by Anderson. Clearly outlining factors related to the etiology, assessment and treatment of substance abuse and dependency in gay men and lesbians, Anderson has pulled together an impressive amount of literature related to this topic and makes informed suggestions for work with this population.

Connolly outlines issues of importance for older gay men and lesbians, and discusses the legal issues that need to be considered within the health care setting. Her case example speaks poignantly to the need for social workers not only to assess the barriers faced within the health care system, but also to the need for clients to be protected after discharge. Ettelbrick continues this discussion, outlining the steps that gay men and lesbians need to take in order to have legal protection in case of serious health problems or death.

The legal issues discussed by Ettelbrick are seen throughout the preceding articles. While all men and women need to voice their medical wishes through a living will, gay men and lesbians must also have legal documents which protect their property rights, and even rights for hospital visitation. Changes in the law which allow gay and lesbian couples the same rights and privileges as heterosexual married couples would alleviate the need for this legal vigilance, as well as insure equal access to health insurance.

Along with legal changes protecting the rights of gay men and lesbians affected by illness, each of the authors speaks to the need for education about sexual orientation to be included in the curriculum of all professional schools. Ignorance of the special needs and issues confronting gay men and lesbians is a major barrier to better treatment within the health care system. Education may be the best way to combat heterosexism, while legal protection is needed against homophobia.

These articles speak specifically to the needs of gay and lesbian people within the health care system. Social workers also need to be aware of the barriers that gay men and lesbians face not only within the health care arena, but also with connecting systems. Social workers need to be knowledgeable about professional resources in their communities where gay men and lesbians can receive services that are of high quality and sensitive to their particular needs. Whether it be lawyers who can help complete the necessary legal documents, or mental health professionals who can work with families, providers in health care need to have these referral sources available.

None of these issues would be important if homophobia and heterosexism were not so rampant in our society. It is hoped that the following articles will help educate readers to some of the issues confronting gay and lesbian people in the health care arena, and that some day every gay man and lesbian will have positive health care experiences.

K. Jean Peterson, DSW

REFERENCES

Douglas, C. J., Kalman, C. M., & Kalman, T. P. (1985). Homophobia among physicians and nurses: An empirical study. *Hospital and Community Psychiatry, 36*(12), 1309-1311.

Robertson, P., & Schachter, J. (1981). Failure to identify venereal disease in a lesbian population. *Sexually Transmitted Diseases, 8*(2), 16-17.

Smith, E. M., Johnson, S. R., & Guenther, S. M. (1985). Health care attitudes and experiences during gynecologic care among lesbians and bisexuals. *American Journal of Public Health, 75*(9), 1085-1087.

Lesbian and Gay Youth
in a Straight World:
Implications for Health Care Workers

Harvey L. Gochros
Robert Bidwell

SUMMARY. Many homosexually oriented youth remain invisible, caught in the struggle between their same sex attractions and need for peer group approval. This article discusses the sub-populations among gay and lesbian youth, as well as the psychological risks, interpersonal stresses, and health risks experienced by this group. Health care providers have a unique opportunity to recognize the special needs of their gay and lesbian adolescent patients, but face formidable barriers to providing these services. However, there are also enormous opportunities for developing innovative and early intervention programs on behalf of gay and lesbian youth. Special issues which need to be considered in developing these programs are discussed. *[Article copies available from The Haworth Document Delivery Service: 1-800-342-9678.]*

Academicians are currently debating whether homosexual orientation is genetic or learned. If indeed a predisposition to homosexuality

---

Harvey L. Gochros, DSW, is Professor, School of Social Work, University of Hawaii-Manoa, 2500 Campus Road, Honolulu, HI 96822. Robert Bidwell, MD, is with the Department of Pediatrics, University of Hawaii Medical School.

[Haworth co-indexing entry note]: "Lesbian and Gay Youth in a Straight World: Implications for Health Care Workers." Gochros, Harvey L., and Robert Bidwell. Co-published simultaneously in *Journal of Gay & Lesbian Social Services* (The Haworth Press, Inc.) Vol. 5, No. 1, 1996, pp. 1-17; and: *Health Care for Lesbians and Gay Men: Confronting Homophobia and Heterosexism* (ed: K. Jean Peterson) The Haworth Press, Inc., 1996, pp. 1-17; and: *Health Care for Lesbians and Gay Men: Confronting Homophobia and Heterosexism* (ed: K. Jean Peterson) Harrington Park Press, an imprint of The Haworth Press, Inc., 1996, pp. 1-17. Single or multiple copies of this article are available from The Haworth Document Delivery Service [1-800-342-9678, 9:00 a.m. - 5:00 p.m. (EST)].

1

is inborn, anticipated advances in genetic engineering raise the specter that some day parents may be in a position to decide whether to abort fetuses that have a homosexual disposing gene.

Whether homosexuality is inborn or acquired, however, there are countless thousands of adolescents who suffer silently as a result of their homosexual feelings, largely because of society's pervasive negative attitudes about same-sex erotic attraction. Like other "alienated" adolescents, lesbian and gay youth experience the negative health consequences that result from isolation, fear, violence and the requisites of day-to-day survival. Health care providers are in an excellent position to address the medical and psychosocial needs of these young people. Indeed, in 1993, the American Academy of Pediatrics officially endorsed the responsibility of pediatric providers to recognize their lesbian and gay patients and to address their special experience and needs (Committee on Adolescence, 1993). Similarly, in 1992 the American Medical Association published its *Guidelines for Adolescent Preventive Services (GAPS)* (American Medical Association, 1992) which set a standard for the routine discussion of sexual orientation on an annual basis with all adolescents.

Unfortunately, there is some evidence suggesting that health providers have abdicated their responsibility to youth at risk. Research indicates that in many health care settings meaningful contact between providers and adolescent patients does not take place. Most provider-patient encounters involve only very brief (14 minutes) and sporadic visits (Nelson, 1991). Furthermore, physicians, social workers and other health providers acknowledge both a lack of training and comfort related to counseling adolescents about substance use, sexual activity and other risk behaviors (Blum & Bearinger, 1990). Research indicates that these issues are not routinely discussed with most teen patients/clients (Joffe, Radius, & Gall, 1988). Adolescents growing up in deprived conditions are less likely to access health care and counseling than other adolescents, although their needs may be greater. Finally, gay and lesbian teenagers will not often reveal their sexual orientation to health providers for fear of censure, and therefore will not receive appropriate medical care and anticipatory guidance (Remafedi & Blum, 1986).

LESBIAN AND GAY YOUTH

Incidence of Homosexual Orientation in Youth

The sexual orientation of adults or youth has not been included in our national census. Even if it were, these data would be difficult to elicit. Indeed, the majority of homosexually and bisexually oriented youth do not label themselves as "gay" or "lesbian" and do not fit the cultural stereotypes of how gay and lesbians appear and behave.

Because of their homophobic environment many of these adolescents hope that their same sex interest is only a transitory phase, or that given the right circumstances (engaging in sexual activities with partners of the other sex, for example) they will be "cured." Even when they do self-label as homosexual or bisexual, they still might choose to deny their sexual interests to others—including sex researchers. These factors contribute to the "invisibility" of this population and make it almost impossible to accurately estimate its size.

To complicate matters further, defining sexual orientation involves more than determining with whom someone shared genital contact. Many studies only report explicit sexual contact with others of the same sex. Sexuality, however, involves more than erotic activities. It includes one's gender identity, the sex of people with whom one has romantic as well as erotic fantasies, and which socially prescribed sex-role behavior one models.

Also, perhaps a third of adolescents experience (and may continue to experience) sexual interests in *both* genders. Young people are usually highly eroticized and at the height of their erotic potential. They may therefore be responsive to a range of sexual stimuli.

Despite these factors, because of contemporary western culture's pressure to bifurcate sexual orientation, many youth experience society's pressure to "make a choice."

Most current estimates, based on limited data, suggest that somewhere between three to ten percent of the population have a predominately homosexual orientation. A larger percentage may be bisexual. Research has often been of limited value since frequently it surveys sexual behaviors rather than other aspects of sexuality such as attraction, fantasy and self-designation as gay or lesbian. Many, if not most, gay and lesbian teenagers have never been sexually active but are acutely aware of their emerging sexual orientation. A recent large-scale survey of Minnesota adolescents found that by age 18, 6.4% of adolescents acknowledge predominately homosexual attractions, although smaller percentages of adolescents had ever been homosexually active or labeled themselves homosexual (Remafedi, Resnick, Blum, & Harris, 1992).

Who Are These Youth?

Most homosexually oriented youth are indistinguishable from other youth aside from the nature of their same-sex interests. Their sexual orientation is usually "invisible" to their teachers, friends and even their own families. Only a minority choose to reveal their sexual orientation even to their closest friends. Their problems are compounded, however, by the fact that in addition to dealing with conflicts associated with their sexual orientation, they also face all the other complex developmental tasks faced by adolescents.

Age of Awareness

The age at which homosexually oriented youth recognize their same sex interest, and the age at which they actually engage in homosexual contacts varies greatly (Troiden, 1988). Surveys find that gay men and lesbians recall the age of their first same-sex activity as approximately 15 years for males and 20 years for females. Self-labeling as "gay" or "lesbian," if it occurs at all, usually comes still later.

Because of their invisibility and the denial these adolescents invoke in response to same sex feelings, many health care professionals underestimate the numbers of homosexually oriented youths and find it difficult to detect and reach troubled youth with whom they come in contact. Consequently, they may fail to initiate or support programs to meet the needs of these youths. The invisibility of these youths also allows homosexually oriented youths to hide their sexual concerns and avoid or delay dealing with the implications and the developmental tasks associated with homosexuality.

Reactions to Homosexual Orientation

Many homosexually oriented youths view their emerging homosexual identity primarily as a loss of their heterosexual potential and all that this entails–loss of status, parental and social disapproval, uncertain civil rights, and possibly the loss of marital and parental potential.

The discomfort with a gay or lesbian orientation could not come at a worse stage of development. Most adolescents are just beginning to develop a sense of identity and self-esteem nurtured by identification with a reference group of peers. Most of their peers are developing heterosexual identities and communicate a preoccupation with successfully making it in a heterosexual world. This can heighten the homosexually oriented youth's sense of difference and non-conformity. It also often removes the opportunity for peer support for any difficulties the homosexually oriented youth might be encountering in her/his sexual development. Some adolescents try to compensate, deny or hide their feared sexual identity by becoming active in sports, participating in anti-gay harassment, seeking heterosexual experiences, or even by producing children.

Special Sub-Populations

Experimenters. Many young people explore same sex activities out of curiosity. Some fear that they may be homosexual and decide to "test it out," especially when they are sexually intimidated by the other gender or are feeling powerful erotic urges when heterosexual outlets are not available. Others pride themselves as risk takers and perceive a homosexual activity as an adventure–not unlike their approach to alcohol, drugs or other potentially risky behaviors.

Bisexual-Ambisexual. Some people grow up with a capacity for attraction to both sexes. They encounter, however, various social forces pressing them to choose. Labeling oneself as bisexual may therefore be a defensive step in the long-term process of "coming out" for some youth.

Ethnic minority and immigrant youth. There is considerable diversity in cultural perceptions and sanctions regarding the acceptable range of sexual behaviors in youth. In some cultures, some degree of homosexual activity is considered natural and of no concern to the adult community. In middle American culture, many adolescents find themselves in the difficult position of being in an oppressed sexual minority (homosexual) within a powerless age minority (youth) within an oppressed ethnic and cultural minority.

The physically and mentally disabled. There is little social recognition or acceptance of the sexuality, let alone homosexuality, of the physically and mentally disabled. The youth in these categories find little support for their evolving sexuality. Health providers as well as parents and other care givers will often block out the possibility of their charges even being sexual. They may have so many other care issues to contend with that sex, let alone homosexuality, would be the last thing on their minds.

Rural youth. Homosexually oriented youth growing up in rural areas are even more isolated than their urban peers. They are likely to have limited interpersonal contacts with other gay and lesbian youths and less access to gay supportive adults, programs or literature.

Transgendered and cross-dressing youths. Youth who perceive themselves as being members of the opposite sex experience an additional layer of oppression, partly because their sexual identity is more visible. These youths not only are considered a threat by their straight peers, but are often rejected by their role "appropriate" gay peers.

RISKS ENCOUNTERED BY HOMOSEXUALLY ORIENTED YOUTH

Homosexually oriented youth encounter numerous risks to their psychological and emotional health, largely as a result of their coping with the attitudes and behaviors of people in their environment. Some of these risks include psychological risks, interpersonal stress, and health risks.

Psychological Risks

Coming out. Homosexually oriented youths are psychologically at risk whether or not they reveal their orientation to others. If they choose to keep their interests secret, as many do, they run the risk of isolation, and depression that often leads to suicide. If they reveal their orientation to family and/or peers they risk rejection, ridicule, hostility and even violence.

Harassment and violence. Widely accepted prejudice toward gays and lesbians makes these youths vulnerable to harassment and physical violence at school and in the community. Many are subjected to hostile homophobic comments not only from classmates but from their teachers as well. Often family members react violently to the homosexual disclosure of an adolescent family member. Violent parental reactions often lead many of these youths to leave home. Indeed, many are forced out of their homes by one or both parents and turn to a life on the streets, often involving drugs and prostitution.

Interpersonal Stress

The loss of peer acceptance can be particularly critical for adolescents who depend on this support in the process of developing their identity and self-esteem. Adolescents with evolving homosexual identities lack many of the critical opportunities and sanctions that are available to heterosexual youths to learn intimacy skills from their contacts with other youths. They pay a high price for being different in a youth culture that calls for conformity. They need a sense of belonging as they make the transition from family identity to individual identity. Like other alienated, rejected and isolated youth they are vulnerable to love and possible exploitation from lesbian and gay adults.

Health Risks

The ignorance, isolation and fear encountered by many gay and lesbian youth can profoundly affect their physical well-being. The following may be considered possible indicators of teenagers dealing with sexual concerns.

Sexually transmitted diseases (STDs). Gay and lesbian youths may be heterosexually active, or sometimes not sexually active at all. Furthermore, there are few practices that are exclusive to the sexual repertoire of gays and lesbians. Exclusively homosexual lesbian teenagers generally experience fewer STDs than their heterosexual peers. They may, however, have vaginitis due to herpes, Trichomonas, Candida and Gardnerella. They may also be at risk for HIV through contact with menstrual blood. The provider should remember that some lesbian youth may be heterosexually active or have a female partner who is, and therefore be at additional risk for gonorrhea, chlamydia, syphilis and genital warts.

Exclusively homosexual gay male teens may contract many of the same STDs as heterosexual males, including gonorrhea and chlamydia. Not all gay male teenagers engage in anal intercourse, but those who do are subject to rectal gonorrhea and chlamydia as well as local trauma to rectal tissue. Syphilis, genital warts, HIV, cytomegalovirus (CMV), hepatitis B and a variety of gastrointestinal infections are also possible. It should be noted that physical complaints or symptoms are a much less reliable screen for sexual orientation than is a careful, confidential and non-judgmental medical and psychosocial history.

Alcohol and other drugs. Alcohol serves to anesthetize and reduce the psychic pain experienced by many adolescents. Further, it serves as a social and sexual psychological lubricant for those who are uncomfortable with their sexuality. Gay and lesbian bars may provide the only outlet to meet other similarly oriented people. Gay and lesbian youth can be reasonably sure that everyone there is gay or lesbian and therefore potential social and sexual contacts.

Sexual distress. As a result of the guilt about their sexuality some homosexually oriented youth develop dysfunctional and inhibited sexual attitudes and behaviors. Sexual orientation concerns also should be considered with any teenager engaged in extensive sexual activity, either homosexual or heterosexual.

Prostitution and sexual/emotional exploitation. Prostitution, with all its associated dangers, is often a product of a gay or lesbian youth's search for love and acceptance from the adult world as well as a basic survival strategy for those living on the streets.

Sequela of denial. Some teenagers actively seek pregnancy in an attempt to deny their homosexual feelings and assert a heterosexual identity in a heterosexist culture. Many will also choose heterosexual marriage for the same reason.

Sequela of violence. Gays and lesbians of all ages are frequently subjected to violent reactions by those who oppose their lifestyles. The most common settings for such attacks on gay and lesbian youths are from classmates in school and even more frequently from parents in their homes. Such violent rejection often leads to truancy and to gay and lesbian youth leaving home. They also frequently encounter aggression from peers in their communities when their orientation is revealed or even suspected. A significant danger of serious physical attacks occurs when they mistakenly make sexual advances to homophobic peers, implicitly suggesting that the peer may be homosexually oriented as well.

Loneliness, depression and suicide. Homosexually oriented youth often lack the opportunities, sanctions and interpersonal skills for developing mutually rewarding intimate relationships. Sexual encounters may sometimes provide frequent but not usually long-lasting palliative relief from their loneliness. Consequently many see nothing but an empty future ahead of them. This pessimism is often reinforced by the lack of any visible "happy" homosexual role models. Without hope, suicide may seem the only option. It appears that among gay male youths those most at risk have more feminine gender roles, have adopted a gay or bisexual identity at an earlier age, and are more likely to have experienced sexual abuse, substance use and arrests for misconduct (Remafedi, Farrow, & Deisher, 1991).

CONTACT WITH THE HEALTH CARE ARENA

Gay and lesbian youth, because they are both physically and psychosocially at risk, are likely to have frequent encounters with the health care arena. This arena is defined in the broadest of terms to include the physical, emotional, psychological, social and spiritual health of adolescents. It includes individual encounters between the professional and patient/client as well as the institutional milieu within the community.

A multidisciplinary approach should be developed to address the needs of individual gay and lesbian youth. In addition, a community-wide network of supportive programs and services (e.g., telephone hotlines, shelters, peer counseling and walk-in crisis centers) should be created. Together, social workers, physicians, nurse practitioners, counselors, teachers, clergy and other youth professionals must work as co-equal partners in developing new programs and refurbishing old programs so that the needs of both "visible" and "invisible" gay and lesbian youth are recognized and addressed. There must also be a recognition that if any link in the community network is missing or weak, youths will be lost or hurt. Models of this sort of community cooperation on the behalf of gay and lesbian youth exist in Seattle, Minneapolis, Washington, D.C., Boston and other cities across the United States.

Barriers

In many communities there have existed profound barriers to the provision of health care to gay and lesbian youth. These barriers have prevented individual professionals from addressing issues of sexual orientation with clients/patients. They have also prevented the development of much needed programs and community-wide networks of services for sexual minority youth.

Lack of knowledge. One of the most fundamental barriers has been the widespread lack of knowledge among youth professionals about the nature of sexual orientation and the issues faced by lesbian and gay youth. Many recognize gay and lesbian youth only when they conform to stereotypes, and do not recognize that the great majority of these teens, perhaps 5 to 10 percent of the general population, is "invisible." They are not aware that many youth experiencing substance use, school and family problems, and runaway or suicidal behaviors may be responding to sexual orientation concerns. Many professionals working with youth are unaware that in many fields, often their own, homosexuality is considered a normal part of the spectrum of human sexuality. They are also unfamiliar with the growing number of model programs that address the needs of these youth and may even be unaware of programs or resources in their own communities.

This lack of knowledge is based, at least in part, in the failure of professional schools to acknowledge the existence and specific needs of sexual minority youth in their curricula. This silence is also seen in the reluctance of youth-service agencies to provide their staff with either the permission or skills to work effectively with this population.

The result has been that myths and stereotypes about homosexuality have been allowed to go unchallenged, despite the growing body of research related to the nature of sexual orientation and the dangers of growing up lesbian and gay in a hostile environment. Services continue to be directed, if at all, only to those youths that fit a stereotype (for example, the cross-dressing male or the street hustler) while ignoring the great majority who are indistinguishable from other teenagers. In a sense, too, this ignorance has allowed HIV/AIDS to dominate any discussion of gay youth when, in fact, the need for recognition, acceptance and support may be as great or greater than the need for HIV/AIDS information or services.

It is likely that many—if not most—health care workers are not homophobic. That is, they experience neither generalized hostility nor fear toward youth who are homosexually oriented. It is likely, however, that many—if not most—are heterosexist in their approach to young people. That is, they anticipate that all youth are heterosexually oriented and behave toward all youths as if they were heterosexual. Other heterosexist health care workers may accept the inevitability of homosexuality in some of their charges but consider it as an unfortunate "second best" sexual "choice."

Heterosexism among health care providers can manifest itself in many subtle ways. For example, asking adolescent girls if they have a boyfriend, not considering oral or anal areas as potential sites for sexual activity or infection in adolescent boys, failing to offer gay-specific advice on HIV risk reduction, or not exploring the possibility of a sexual identity conflict as the source of suicidal attempts.

To avoid the risks of heterosexism in their practice, health care providers must discard the myth that all youths are heterosexually oriented and the assumption that all homosexually oriented youth conform in appearance or behavior to cultural stereotypes. They must keep in mind the distinct possibility that any youth they encounter in their practice may be experiencing homosexual desires and conflicts.

Fear. A second barrier to providing services and programs for sexual minority youth is the fear experienced by youth professionals, agencies and teens themselves. Individual counselors fear their own lack of knowledge and expertise and the possibility of influencing a confused teen to move toward a homosexual orientation. They also fear negative client/patient, parent or agency reaction, and the loss of job security or a collegial working environment. Perhaps greatest of all is the fear that their own sexual orientation may be called into question. Agencies often fear negative reaction by conservative segments of the community, funding sources and within their own boards of directors if they were to address controversial issues. The question of professional liability in working with gay and lesbian youth is sometimes raised as well.

Teens who may be dealing with sexual orientation concerns may fear accessing existing resources. They may fear being labeled deviant, criminal or sinful. They also fear that any disclosures they might make will not be kept confidential.

These fears have serious implications both programmatically and in individual youth counseling. Important life-saving health issues cannot be addressed if both parties are afraid to approach issues of sexuality in general and sexual orientation in particular. Fear prevents potential advocates from proposing the development of supportive programs at agency planning meetings, community conferences, and legislative hearings. It also means that existing supportive programs or individuals are unknown to the broader community, or if they are known they are not utilized for fear of controversy and reprisals.

Specialization and fragmentation. A third barrier to meeting the needs of lesbian and gay youth is a problem common to the broader adolescent population and the health care arena. This is the tendency of programs and disciplines to define their roles narrowly rather than to view them as overlapping and complementary. Thus, the physician may screen an openly homosexual teen for sexually transmitted diseases (STDs), but not screen for suicidal ideation. The social worker may discuss suicidal ideation, but not address specific sexual behaviors and the risk of HIV or other STDs. The probation officer may monitor a young person's truancy or runaway activity, but not advocate for gay/lesbian friendly foster home placement options in the community. These narrow perspectives result in fragmented care and inhibit the creation of networks of supportive services and programs.

Community values. A fourth barrier lies in unsupportive, even oppressive, community values related to minority sexual orientations in some communities. These attitudes often arise from, though are not limited to, conservative religious traditions that view sexual activity outside of the procreative sphere as dirty or sinful. While they may not reflect majority community opinion, the vociferousness with which these beliefs are presented in the pulpit, in the media, and at community forums such as school board meetings, creates a great deal of fear among agencies that may understand the needs of lesbian and gay youth but wish to avoid controversy or censure.

These barriers do not exist in isolation. Ignorance, fear, narrowly defined roles and oppressive community attitudes often reinforce each other in preventing the development of needed services and programs for sexual minority youth.

Opportunities

Despite the many formidable barriers to creating a health care arena that is responsive to the needs of lesbian and gay youth, there probably never before have been such enormous opportunities for creating innovative programs and early intervention strategies on their behalf.

Perhaps most important in this regard is the clear movement in American society over the past 40 years toward greater acceptance of gay, lesbian and bisexual people. Public dialogue about issues of sexual orientation occurs today that never took place two generations ago. Although this dialogue has been slow to extend to youth issues, in the past five years there have been increasing numbers of local and national conferences and policy statements by youth professional organizations related to sexual minority youth. This activity has been bolstered by the knowledge coming from continuing research into the nature and origins of sexual orientation and more recently by studies documenting the experience of growing up gay or lesbian in American society.

More and more youth agencies and health organizations across the country have begun to provide in-service training to their staff on gay youth issues. In several communities, such as Seattle, networks of youth service agencies, schools and religion-affiliated groups have been developed to conduct needs assessments and coordinate community-wide program development for both "visible" and "invisible" gay and lesbian youth. These model networks demonstrate how coalitions of diverse agencies can be created and also show that mainline "respectable" agencies can address controversial issues without community censure or loss of funding. In fact, what many agencies have discovered is that funding is available when credible agencies put forth creative, even provocative, proposals related to sexual minority youth. These models can provide great reassurance to other communities taking their first steps in network building.

PROGRAM DEVELOPMENT

How can youth agencies, schools and individual youth professionals take advantage of this new climate of openly addressing gay youth issues? Many have taken steps to increase their awareness of and sensitivity to gay and lesbian youth (and staff) within their individual agencies. This has meant instituting formal and regular in-service training of administrative, supervisory and front-line staff on what is now known about sexual orientation and the experience of growing up lesbian or gay. This includes recognizing that 5 to 10 percent of students or clients may be dealing with an emerging gay or lesbian identity. Staff should recognize that these young people cannot be reliably identified through stereotypes. Sexual orientation should be addressed routinely in health screening interviews with *all* adolescents, since few teenagers will independently acknowledge sexual orientation concerns.

After appropriate assurances of confidentiality, and in the context of a broader social history, the health provider can ask, "Have you ever dated or gone steady with anyone?" This should be followed by "Have you ever had sex with another person?" If yes, ask "Have your partners been males, females or both?" If the teenager acknowledges sexual activity of any kind, the interviewer should determine frequency, kinds of sexual activity, kinds of partners (friends or anonymous), where sexual activity occurs, whether the encounters are voluntary or coerced, or whether there has been an exchange of money or drugs for sex. A history of pregnancy or STDs should also be obtained, as well as any history of substance use, family or peer conflict, or suicidal ideation.

The interview should also address whether patients/clients consider themselves to be gay or lesbian and, if so, the degree of distress this causes them. Many gay and lesbian teenagers are not yet sexually active but have experienced significant distress as they recognize their emerging orientation. The health provider should say, "Some of the teens I work with have feelings of attraction to members of the same sex. This is perfectly natural but can worry some teens a lot. I'm wondering if you have ever had these kinds of feelings or worries." The gay teenager may or may not be able to acknowledge such feelings, but the message has been given that they are not alone and that there is someone to talk to when the time is right for them. Finally, it is important to learn if teenagers have support systems to help them during their "coming out" process.

Any youth who has considered suicide, turned to drugs, or had problems at home or school may well be someone struggling with important issues related to sexual orientation. The role of schools, agencies and counselors is not to label these youths as gay or lesbian. Instead, they can help a young person examine his or her experiences and feelings, including sexual orientation, and provide information, correct misconceptions and facilitate access to supportive community services, such as medical care and teen support groups for lesbian and gay youth.

Some individuals and agencies that are somewhat uncomfortable about openly addressing sexual orientation issues have developed a position that the programs they have created are not endorsing a particular sexual orientation but simply addressing a reality–that some youth identify themselves, or are identified by others, as gay or lesbian, and that research has shown that bad things often happen to these young people.

In addition to training, some agencies have found it important to develop mission statements and policies that specifically mention sexual minority youth as among those served. They state that it is not only permitted, but also expected that staff will develop services and work individually with clients/students in an open and forth-right manner on issues related to sexual orientation.

Specific program content will vary from agency to agency and will depend on the extent to which a community network exists. Optimally, all youth agencies, programs and schools will be in a position to provide information and dispel myths and misconceptions about homosexuality through books, brochures and counseling. Very concrete, visible and specific messages should be given teen clients/patients through posters or brochures that concerns or confusion about sexual orientation can be discussed in a confidential and supportive manner with designated staff. Clearly, agency consent and confidentiality issues must be examined to determine whether the agency is teen-accessible in this regard. It is fortunate that the trend has been toward recognizing greater adolescent autonomy in giving consent for health care services.

The community-wide networks that are created to provide support for sexual minority youth should go beyond targeting youth already "visible" or engaged in high-risk behaviors. They must provide protection, information and anticipating guidance for all youth with sexual orientation concerns, including the majority of gay and lesbian teens who may be isolated and confused but not involved with drugs or street life and who are not yet sexually active. For example, the time for providing preventive services such as hepatitis B immunization, instruction in condom/dental dam usage and so forth, is before sexual activity has begun.

These networks are effective only if they include the active participation of schools, youth agencies, health centers, the religious community and the media, and provide a mechanism for ongoing needs assessment and strategic planning to fill gaps in services. These networks might include public and private agencies and organizations that provide gay/lesbian-sensitive foster homes, teen hotlines, speakers' bureaus, training, support groups geographically accessible throughout the community, theater workshops for youth, city and school library teen reading lists, city or agency sponsored dances, film nights and other social events. These networks might also develop multi-service, multi-agency sponsored drop-in centers for sexual minority youth.

Perhaps most importantly, this network can serve as an advocate and educator throughout the community on the importance and responsibility of meeting the needs of all youth, including lesbian and gay adolescents.

CONCLUSION

The adolescent years can be marked by very real dangers as well as great opportunities for self-discovery and growth. This is as true for gay and lesbian teens as it is for their heterosexual peers. Nevertheless, the experience of sexual minority youth is a special one. Most are "invisible" and carry with them a "hidden secret" with its attendant guilt, and both realistic and unrealistic fears. The health care arena, in its broadest definition, can play an important role in reducing the risks and enhancing growth. It can only do this if it is willing to accept controversy and openly and comprehensively address the realities of gay and lesbian youth.

REFERENCES

American Medical Association (1992). *Guidelines for adolescent preventive services (GAPS)*. Chicago, IL: American Medical Association.

Blum, R. W., & Bearinger, L. (1990). Knowledge and attitudes of health professionals toward adolescent health care. *Journal of Adolescent Health Care*, *11*(4), 289-94.

Committee on Adolescence, American Academy of Pediatrics (1993). Homosexuality and adolescence. *Pediatrics*, *92*(4), 631-34.

Joffe, A., Radius, S., & Gall, M. (1988). Health counseling for adolescents: What they want, what they get, and who gives it. *Pediatrics*, *82*(3 Pt 2), 481-85.

Nelson, C. (1991, April 11). *Advance data from vital and health statistics of the national center for health statistics* (DHHS Publication No. 196). Washington, DC: U.S. Government Printing Office.

Remafedi, G., & Blum, R. (1986). Working with gay and lesbian adolescents. *Pediatric Annals*, *15*(11), 773-83.

Remafedi, G., Farrow, J., & Deisher, R. (1991). Risk factors for attempted suicide in gay and bisexual youth. *Pediatrics*, *87*(6), 869-75.

Remafedi, G., Resnick, M., Blum, R., & Harris, L. (1992). Demography of sexual orientation in adolescents. *Pediatrics*, *89*(4 Pt 2), 714-21.

Troiden, R. R. (1988). Homosexual identity development. *Journal of Adolescent Health Care*, *9*(2), 105-13.

Gay Men and the Health Care System

Martin Schwartz

SUMMARY. Because of the homophobia manifested by health care providers, gay men have had to exercise extra prudence in the selection of their physician to avoid "second class" medical care. The persistence of negative attitudes of caretakers towards gay men is evident in the interaction between the physician and her/his gay male patient. These negative attitudes are manifested in a range of behaviors, from overt rejection to benign neglect. To avoid this deleterious experience, some gay men will withhold pertinent information which subsequently interferes with the physician's ability to make an appropriate diagnosis. The AIDS epidemic has led to a confrontation of the health system by gay activists and AIDS service organizations, ushering in the start of more positive attitudes and behaviors towards gay men with HIV or AIDS. Possible solutions to these shameful occurrences with the health system are discussed. *[Article copies available from The Haworth Document Delivery Service: 1-800-342-9678.]*

HOMOPHOBIA AND HEALTH CARE PROVIDERS

John has been dealing with his inner homophobia ever since he acknowledged his gay sexual orientation and sexual identi-

Martin Schwartz, EdD, BCD, LCSW, is affiliated with Virginia Commonwealth University School of Social Work, 1001 West Franklin Street, Box 2027, Richmond, VA 23284-2027.

[Haworth co-indexing entry note]: "Gay Men and the Health Care System." Schwartz, Martin. Co-published simultaneously in *Journal of Gay & Lesbian Social Services* (The Haworth Press, Inc.) Vol. 5, No. 1, 1996, pp. 19-32; and: *Health Care for Lesbians and Gay Men: Confronting Homophobia and Heterosexism* (ed: K. Jean Peterson) The Haworth Press, Inc., 1996, pp. 19-32; and: *Health Care for Lesbians and Gay Men: Confronting Homophobia and Heterosexism* (ed: K. Jean Peterson) Harrington Park Press, an imprint of The Haworth Press, Inc., 1996, pp. 19-32. Single or multiple copies of this article are available from The Haworth Document Delivery Service [1-800-342-9678, 9:00 a.m. - 5:00 p.m. (EST)].

ty. He sought therapy as he recognized that he was restricting his interpersonal and sexual life to the point that he was isolated and lonely. Manifestations of his shame and guilt about his homosexuality were evident in his irrational anxieties about being infected with HIV as well as symptoms of impotency. Because of the latter, John was referred to a urologist to determine if there was any physical basis for the inability to maintain an erection. Masturbation was the only way that John could gain some sexual pleasure without resulting anxiety. The lack of erections was not only frustrating to John, but the absence of any sexual pleasure often left him depressed.

John reported that the urologist's demeanor changed from an overt expression of concern for John and his psychological pain to a complete dismissal of his difficulties when John informed the doctor that he was gay. In essence, the physician's message was that the impotency was a fitting retribution for John's homosexuality. There was no physical workup nor any future appointment made.

There is no doubt that this transaction would have been different if John was heterosexual. Failure to achieve a full erection is one of the more momentous insults to the male ego and the medical profession has responded accordingly, utilizing its knowledge and technology to treat male impotence. In John's case, the homophobia of the urologist interfered with his commitment to the Hippocratic oath. Sadly, John's transaction with the physician is not atypical. Gay men have had to deal with homophobia in an arena where trust, confidence, acceptance and caring are crucial elements of the helping relationship. Homophobia by health care providers is manifested in a range of reactions, from overt rejection, to benign neglect of gay male patients.

This "second class" status is avoided by many gay men by not sharing their sexual identity, reinforcing their internalized homophobia and belief that their gayness is unacceptable. In addition, the ability of the physician to make appropriate diagnoses is hampered by the patient withholding any information he perceives will identify him as gay. A devastating result of this secrecy may be inappropriate treatment which will negatively affect the gay male's health and survival. It is criminal to consider that a patient turning to the professional for succor, seeking release from pain as well as human understanding, is denied this intervention simply because he is gay. It is abominable to think that a young, gay adolescent seeking information about his budding sexuality from an "informed" medical adult could experience a humiliating lecture about the evil of his sexual orientation.

While homophobia and the "second class" status of gay men have always been present in the health care system, they have become even more blatant with the AIDS epidemic. Scherer, Wu, and Haughey (1991) among others (Fikar, 1992; Kelly, St. Lawrence, Smith, & Cook, 1987) have found that among physicians there is a direct correlation between negative attitudes towards gay men and lesbians and an unwillingness to care for homosexuals with AIDS. The AIDS epidemic has created a shock wave throughout the health system and the health professional's "usual" noxious treatment of gay men infected with HIV has clashed with an assertive demand by gay men and AIDS service organizations that this is no longer tolerable.

In the beginning of the AIDS epidemic, the treatment of gay men with AIDS was a clear manifestation of the system's homophobia. The rejection, isolation and prejudiced responses of society, who perceived gay men with HIV as lepers who were now being punished for their aberrant behavior, was manifested in the health system's policies and treatment of gay men infected with HIV:

> Many health-care professionals themselves treated the AIDS patients worse than leprosy patients, often keeping them waiting for hours until they passed out in a little side room, where they had been placed and then forgotten. They would wear masks and gowns just to talk to them or they would sit five feet away from them while getting information. When one of the patients wanted to make a phone call, the nurse screamed at him, "don't you touch that phone," and then scrubbed it as if he had vomited on it. (Kubler-Ross, 1988, p. 20)

Current research shows that ignorance about HIV (Peterson, 1992) and negative attitudes still exist among health care professionals (Bernstein, Rabkin, & Wolland, 1990; Currey, Johnson, &

Ogden, 1990). There are doctors, dentists and allied health professionals who will not attend HIV and AIDS clients. A survey of physicians and dentists in Virginia found that although most physicians reported being well-informed about AIDS, nearly a third of those questioned said they were unwilling or somewhat unwilling to treat patients infected with the deadly virus. This same survey found that 70 percent of 522 Virginia dentists surveyed are unwilling or somewhat unwilling to treat people infected with the AIDS virus (Orndoff, 1988).

Changes have taken place, albeit at a slow pace. Overt rejection has been replaced with a professional caring of some gay men with HIV and AIDS. There is greater acceptance of gay relationships, and the patient's significant other is more often treated as a legitimate family member. The AIDS activist groups have forced significant changes in the procedures of testing new drugs which have saved thousands of gay men's lives. However, it should be noted that these changes have taken place with a small number of health professionals, predominately those who have been actively involved in serving HIV and AIDS clients. The battle against homophobia in the health system continues (Emanuel, 1988).

While AIDS activists are waging war against prejudice and discrimination of persons infected with the HIV virus, the individual gay male contends with the immediate impact of homophobia alone. From selecting a physician, to deciding what to disclose, the gay male must contend with issues that reflect both homophobia and heterosexism.

Selection of a Physician

Our television sets tell us that the selection of our personal doctor is a very private decision and that there are doctors who are concerned, well-trained specialists who are awaiting our call to set up an appointment. In fact, there are organizations in the community which will provide us with the "right" kind of doctor for our particular difficulties. Does a gay male, new to the community, contact this community service to inquire which physician is gay or gay-accepting? In most instances the answer is an emphatic "No," and even if asked there is doubt the information would be available to the caller. Yet, the issue is pivotal for the gay male as long as anti-gay attitudes exist among health care providers. The gay male must carefully select his primary care physician. In this relationship, the gay male seeks an expert on medical matters whose advice and counsel are guided by the physician's acumen, not his/her prejudice. Furthermore, the gay male does not want to experience shame, negative judgment and rejection from the very person he has gone to for aid. The gay male wants a professional who can accept him wholly and one for whom his sexual identity is not the critical element in determining the transaction between him and his physician.

What are his choices? The gay male can decide that his preference is someone who is convenient, reputable, accessible, and most importantly, a doctor whose specialization is congruent with his patient's medical needs. His selection is swayed by the desire to have an expert. The burning question, which is not answered, is: will this physician be gay-accepting and if not, will the gay male accept the negative consequences of this selection? Can he rationalize that his gayness will never become a factor in their encounters? He must realize that there are not any legal or professional authorities to whom he can turn if he experiences homophobic attitudes.

Or, the gay male can attempt to find a gay, or gay-accepting physician identified by the gay community or his gay network. Hopefully, this doctor also has the medical expertise he needs. Certainly, this selection avoids the unpleasantness and risk of the unknown. Moreover, the gay or gay-accepting doctor's knowledge of the local medical community should prove beneficial should there be a need for referral or hospitalization. But realistically, this option is not available in many communities. It is reprehensible to consider that gay men are forced to go through these machinations to avoid derisive situations because of the existence of irrational attitudes toward homosexuality.

There are also medical emergencies where there is not the time or opportunity to choose the "right" doctor or medical facility.

A client had to be taken to the emergency room by his lover as the client had suddenly fainted while dining out. While awaiting the emergency room physician, the couple experienced continuous belittling comments which caused them to leave without receiving any medical consultation.

For gay men with HIV, selection of a physician is even more critical. They require a caretaker who is *au courant* with the state of knowledge about HIV and opportunistic diseases, and who will treat them with respect and consideration; not a doctor whose ministrations are laden with invalidating attitudes. An AIDS patient stated,

> The doctor I went to formerly simply prescribed medication and didn't necessarily tell me why, or what the side effects might be, or what the end result might be. Any of these things. And if I didn't ask those questions, he would not give me the answers. He wouldn't volunteer, so there was a conspiracy, in effect, of silence.

The physician is often utilized by gay men with HIV as a counselor with whom it is safe to discuss ethical and medical decisions which affect their ability to cope with living with HIV or AIDS. Gay acceptance is an essential component in this relationship.

To Share or Not to Share

To be able to make an appropriate medical diagnosis, the health care provider relies not only on objective measures but on the subjective historical narrative of his/her patient.

> Bill, in a therapy session, complained about a rectal fissure which was interfering with his sex life. He was hesitant to discuss his medical condition with his doctor because of feelings of shame about his sexual practices. Part of his response was due to his own internalized homophobia, which galvanized his fears of others (the doctor and staff) knowing about his homosexuality. Bill did not tell his physician about his sexual practices, and subsequently the physician did not feel Bill needed any medical intervention. Bill preferred to live with the physical discomfort of the rectal fissures, rather than risk the pain of being found out. Later, he went to another physician who operated on him, leaving Bill with an obvious

scar. In a postoperative discussion with Bill, the operating physician joked about how lucky Bill was that he was not gay. Discussion of the symbolic scar and Bill's self-hatred for not asserting himself was a central theme of his work in therapy for some time.

Dealing with the physician is similar to the coming out process that gay men experience all their lives. Each encounter requires a decision about what, if anything, they will share with health care providers. It is difficult for a gay male to discuss his sexual and physical intimacies with another male whose demeanor and outlook communicate repugnance. The gay male cannot anticipate that his physician is familiar with homosexual sexual practices. The physician may be puzzled and perplexed when the patient has some tears in his anus or has been using a "cock" and/or "nipple" ring which has caused some irritation. The unknowing physician may well be astounded if his/her patient discusses the possibility of having his foreskin reinstated or wants to have a medical opinion about some sex toys and paraphernalia used by gay men. If the gay male has become infected with a venereal disease located in his anus, he becomes apprehensive about sharing this with his doctor as he cannot anticipate a nonjudgmental reaction. To escape condemnation, the gay male may feign complete innocence and bewilderment as to the location of the infection.

In his quest for appropriate medical intervention, the gay male should be able to reveal his sexual identity and share any intimate information which will enhance his medical treatment, within a non-homophobic environment.

The Impact of AIDS

One of the more malevolent side effects of the AIDS epidemic has been society's identifying all gay men as carriers of HIV. It has been noted that the increase in gay bashing and legislation depriving gay men and lesbians of their civil rights is related to the overall rejection of this population. AIDS has given people permission to act out their irrational fears and hatred of homosexuals. In addition, the illogical and unscientific attitudes toward the transmission of HIV compound the negative attitude toward gay clients.

Some professionals in the health system have taken the opportunity to exclude gay men from their practices, or assume a posture of benign neglect which communicates clearly that the gay male is not welcome. Should a gay male make it to the office, under these circumstances, he may wonder if he will receive the full attention the situation warrants because of the doctor's reluctance to become involved with a carrier of the virus.

> Robert went to see his dentist at the advice of his AIDS physician as the latter was concerned about Robert's gums (a common disruptive dental problem with HIV-infected individuals). Robert went to his family dentist who had been treating Robert since he was 6 years old. Robert decided to inform his dentist about his HIV status even though the dentist had been practicing universal safety procedures. With much regret, the dentist informed Robert that he could no longer remain a patient in the dentist's practice. The dentist displaced his unethical decision on the fact that his employees, who were mostly women with children, would quit if Robert continued to be a patient in the dentist's practice.

The HIV-positive gay male's need for medical services is critical to his survival. He turns to health care providers not only in medical emergencies, but at times when he is dealing with an opportunistic disease or for preventative prophylaxis treatments. In the beginning of the AIDS epidemic, most physicians were reluctant to become involved with such patients, fearing for their own lives or that their practices would disappear if other patients learned that he/she was treating an HIV patient. In many communities around the country, persons with HIV could not count on their local doctors to either be accepting of them, or knowledgeable about the course of HIV and AIDS.

Presently the response of health care providers is a mixed bag. Women may go undiagnosed as many physicians are not sensitized to the warning signals of HIV in women. Many professionals in the health system do not come in contact with substance abusers. In the first decade it has been the gay male with HIV who has had the most frequent interactions with the health care system and who has led the struggle to demand changes in the system's response to HIV. In spite of numerous educational activities designed to neutralize the irrational fears of health care providers, unnecessary stress on gay men with HIV and AIDS still exists. People with AIDS need caregivers who do not make moral judgments about them (Shalit, 1989).

> Marc, a client with AIDS, went to the hospital pharmacy to pick up his AZT. When the pharmacist told him that queers and faggots who have AIDS need to sit in an isolated section of the waiting room, Marc was identified as a leper for being gay and having the HIV virus. Marc followed the demeaning instructions, stifling his rage because he needed his medication immediately. Some weeks later, through the help of group members, he confronted the pharmacist and the hospital administration who merely censured the pharmacist.

Rejection and discrimination are exacerbated when confidentiality is violated. Confidentiality is a sacrosanct tenet in all professional activities. Unfortunately, its violation has caused many gay men with the HIV virus a great deal of psychological pain, frustration and anger. All patients have the right to expect that the confidentiality of the doctor-patient relationship will be violated only if there are compelling reasons. Lamentably, violations have occurred with little respect for this all-important principle. Clients with HIV have recounted innumerable incidents when their HIV status has "leaked" to receptionists, clerks and bookkeepers who have no medical reason to be informed of their medical diagnosis. The problem is compounded because of the adverse attitudes towards the person who is infected with HIV.

> Sid was HIV positive but asymptomatic. He had been seeing his local physician in conjunction with an AIDS specialist. Sid went in for a routine checkup and was greeted with coolness and disparaging comments by the receptionist who usually was quite warm and friendly to Sid. When Sid went to have his blood pressure taken he was accosted by a nurse in a white gown, mask and rubber gloves. He was told by the nurse that she was protecting herself from being exposed to "that despicable disease you have."

Florence Nightingale would not have approved of the nurse's behaviors nor her acrimonious attitude. This violation of confidentiality can also result in violence.

> Bob was a young adolescent in a residential treatment center when he was diagnosed HIV positive. Three days later he was severely beaten by his peers who attempted to tattoo the word AIDS on his forehead. The standard procedure in that center was that only medical and therapeutic staff should be informed of the adolescent's positive HIV status. Obviously, the information was divulged to the other adolescents.

This "second coming out process," whether by individual choice or unethical professional practice, places gay men with HIV and AIDS in a precarious position. To tell the provider about HIV is an invitation for rejection at many levels.

> Indeed, to get AIDS is precisely to be revealed, in the majority of cases so far, as a member of a certain risk group, a community of pariahs. The illness flushes out an identity that might have remained hidden from neighbors, job mates, family and friends. It also confirms an identity and, among the risk group in the United States most severely affected in the beginning, homosexual men, has been a creator of community as well as an experience that isolates the ill and exposes them to harassment and persecution. (Sontag, 1988, p. 25)

Not to tell the provider about one's HIV status leads to ethical and moral dilemmas. All of this could be eradicated if members of the health system would practice medicine and not discrimination.

> Phil's doctor stayed with him throughout the night that Phil died to make certain that Phil was without pain and receiving appropriate medical care. Prior to this, Phil's physician had made house calls as Phil was too weak to go to the doctor's office. It had been Phil's wish not to die in the hospital, therefore his doctor made all the arrangements to grant Phil's desire.

Clearly, there are professionals in the health system who personify genuine professionalism and human concern.

GAY COUPLES AND THE HEALTH SYSTEM

The negation of the gay couple as a legitimate dyad is glaringly exemplified by the withholding of health insurance benefits by most employers to a gay partner. In addition to discrimination, the couple is faced with the extra financial burden of maintaining two health insurance policies. If one of the couple is unemployed or employed where health insurance is not part of employee benefits, the financial burden can be prohibitive. Moreover, gay couples are often denied the usual amenities granted family members when an illness strikes and/or if there is a need for hospitalization. The healthy member of the couple may not be informed about the diagnosis, prognosis, or course of treatment. While paradoxical, confidentiality may be utilized by the physician as the reason for withholding information, hampering the couple's ability to cope with the impact of the illness together. Even such expected family rights as visiting beyond the usual hours, partaking in the nursing care of the patient, and being able to be with the patient in particularly difficult times is not extended to the gay partner. In the AIDS epidemic, gay couples have fought to have their decisions about invasive medical treatments followed by health care providers. This can be an extremely difficult issue if the patient's family of origin takes a different position from the gay partner. Sometimes, even legal papers are not enough to guarantee the gay couple's wishes. The health care system may question who has the most legitimate legal authority, and decide to support the family of origin rather than the gay family.

> Evan was dying of AIDS when he was hospitalized by his lover, Bruce. The latter notified Evan's family who appeared the next day. Within a few minutes of their arrival, Bruce was informed by the attending physician that he could no longer stay with Evan and that he, the doctor, would follow whatever instructions the family gave him regarding maintaining Evan's life. The family had informed the doctor that Bruce had se-

duced Evan into the deviant lifestyle of homosexuality and that Bruce should be banned from visiting Evan. Bruce was not permitted to say goodbye to his mate nor was he part of the funeral.

PROPOSED SOLUTIONS

Local, state and national gay organizations must be informed of unethical medical practices in order to have the ammunition to wage war on all political levels, and challenge inadequate and unprofessional treatment of gay male clients within the health care system. At the same time, there should be attempts to use the legal system to force changes within the health care system and with health care providers, and greater efforts made to enact a federal bill that guarantees the civil rights of gay men and lesbians.

As suggested earlier, the inner homophobia in gay men contributes not only to a poor self-concept but leads to an invisible, passive stance to prejudiced health care providers' unfair practices. This phenomenon must be dealt with on two levels. First, gay organizations need to initiate support groups for gay men to enhance a positive gay self-concept. Perhaps then, gay men will be more willing to disclose their sexual orientation, thus forcing health care providers to be cognizant of the needs of gay men. Support groups concentrating on gay men's self-esteem can be as effective today in reducing internalized homophobia as they were vital to bringing information, healing and direction to the gay communities in the early years of the AIDS epidemic. Second, gay organizations must increase their public relations efforts to offset anti-gay societal attitudes which still appear to be omnipresent. For example, a recent article in *Time* magazine reported that

when Americans were polled by TIME/CNN last week, about 65% thought homosexual rights were being paid too much attention. Strikingly, those who described homosexuality as morally wrong made up exactly the same proportion–53%–as in a poll in 1978, before a decade of intense gay activism. (Henry, 1994, p. 56)

Continuing efforts to eradicate homophobia from society are imperative to improving the responsiveness of the health care system to the needs of gay men.

Further strategies for eliminating societal homophobia need to include the training and education of all allied health professions as well as the medical and dental professions. Courses on the normal development of the gay male and lesbian female, and content on gay and lesbian couple relationships should be in all graduate professional schools, as well as in mandatory continuing education workshops for *all* health care providers. To achieve the goal of eradicating homophobia, these courses must focus on attitudes, not just information. If possible, the teachers and trainers should be gay or lesbian health professionals.

In addition, gay men and lesbians should serve on the boards of all health agencies (i.e., hospital, clinics, etc.), including health professional regulatory boards to insure that there are no anti-gay practices and that gay men's complaints will be heard.

Finally, it is critical that non-gay men join gay men in the battle to force the health system to be more responsive to gay male patients. When there is a coalition of gay and non-gay men, it is more difficult for those in power to enunciate who is "bad," and who is "good," reducing the ability to divide and conquer. The history of the AIDS epidemic is replete with victories due to the coalition of seropositive and seronegative men and women. Furthermore, the reality is that non-gay men are often in more powerful positions within and outside the health care system than are gay men. As allies, non-gay men can utilize their power and influence to force changes in the health care system.

CONCLUSION

Blatant homophobia, heterosexism, inadequate knowledge and discrimination within the health care system are common experiences for gay men. Even though these barriers have long been present, the advent of AIDS has pointed out their negative impact on the health care of gay men. In addition to these external barriers which gay men face are the internal barriers of fear and internalized homophobia. In order for gay men to receive adequate health care, both of these issues must be confronted. Health care providers need to become aware and knowledgeable about the unique needs of gay men, while gay men must become comfortable in asserting their right to receive appropriate and gay-affirming health care services.

REFERENCES

Bernstein, C. A., Rabkin, J. G., & Wolland, H. (1990). Medical and dental students' attitudes about the AIDS epidemic. *Academic Medicine, 65*(7), 458-460.

Currey, C. J., Johnson, M., & Ogden, B. (1990). Willingness of health professionals to treat patients with AIDS. *Academic Medicine, 65*(7), 472-474.

Emanuel, E. (1988). Do physicians have an obligation to treat patients with AIDS? *New England Journal of Medicine, 318*(25), 1686-1690.

Fikar, C. R. (1992). The gay pediatrician. *Journal of Homosexuality, 23*(3), 53-63.

Henry, W. A., III (1994, June 27). Pride and prejudice. *Time, 143*(26), 54-59.

Kelly, J. A., St. Lawrence, J. S., Smith, S., Jr., & Cook, D. J. (1987). Stigmatization of AIDS patients by physicians. *American Journal of Public Health, 77*(7), 789-791.

Kubler-Ross, E. (1988). *AIDS, the ultimate challenge.* New York: Macmillan.

Orndoff, B. (1988, December 16). Survey of health professionals finds some wary of AIDS cases. *Richmond News Leader*, p. 2.

Peterson, K. J. (1992). Social workers' knowledge about AIDS: Working with vulnerable and oppressed people. *Health and Social Work, 17*(2), 116-127.

Scherer, Y., Wu, Y. W., & Haughey, B. P. (1991). AIDS and homophobia among nurses. *Journal of Homosexuality, 21*(4), 17-27.

Shalit, P. (1989). Jewish law and obligation of the treating physician to heal patients with AIDS. *Journal of American Medical Association, 261*(15), 2199.

Sontag, S. (1988). *AIDS and its metaphors.* New York: Farrar, Straus and Giroux.

Lesbians and the Health Care System

K. Jean Peterson
Mary Bricker-Jenkins

SUMMARY. Lesbians remain invisible within the health care system and have fewer contacts with health care providers. This article reviews the limited research available on health care for lesbians, including the research on the attitudes of health care providers towards lesbians, the health care seeking behavior of lesbians, and the barriers lesbians encounter in seeking care. The experience of lesbians with breast cancer is used to exemplify these issues. Social workers must evaluate and challenge their own attitudes, beliefs, and behaviors if they are to work with, and advocate for, lesbians within the health care system. Recommendations for practice are discussed. *[Article copies available from The Haworth Document Delivery Service: 1-800-342-9678.]*

Only in the past few years has the dearth of research about health care for women been acknowledged as a problem. It was not until 1991 that the new Director of the National Institutes of Health, Bernadine Healy, proposed the Women's Health Initiative and called for women to be included in future health care research

---

K. Jean Peterson, DSW, is Associate Professor, School of Social Welfare, University of Kansas, Lawrence, KS 66045-2510.

Mary Bricker-Jenkins, DSW, is Associate Professor, Department of Social Work, University of Western Kentucky.

[Haworth co-indexing entry note]: "Lesbians and the Health Care System." Peterson, K. Jean, and Mary Bricker-Jenkins. Co-published simultaneously in *Journal of Gay & Lesbian Social Services* (The Haworth Press, Inc.) Vol. 5, No. 1, 1996, pp. 33-47; and: *Health Care for Lesbians and Gay Men: Confronting Homophobia and Heterosexism* (ed: K. Jean Peterson) The Haworth Press, Inc., 1996, pp. 33-47; and: *Health Care for Lesbians and Gay Men: Confronting Homophobia and Heterosexism* (ed: K. Jean Peterson) Harrington Park Press, an imprint of The Haworth Press, Inc., 1996, pp. 33-47. Single or multiple copies of this article are available from The Haworth Document Delivery Service [1-800-342-9678, 9:00 a.m. - 5:00 p.m. (EST)].

33

(Rennie, 1993). However, while the invisibility of women in health care research has finally been acknowledged, the diversity among women requires continued care and vigilance lest invisibility remains for lesbians (White & Levinson, 1993). For example, breast cancer in women has been characterized as a national epidemic, with one-in-eight of all women in the United States being diagnosed with this disease during their lifetime. A recent study by Dr. Suzanne Haynes, a National Cancer Institute (NCI) epidemiologist, suggests that the risk for a lesbian developing breast cancer in her lifetime may be as high as one-in-three (Brownworth, 1993). However, a Medline computer search of juried publications from 1986 to the present found *no* medical studies which looked specifically at breast cancer and lesbians, underscoring the invisibility of lesbians. Lesbians are subsumed either under the category of "women," with no distinctions made based on sexual orientation or as "homosexual," where sexual orientation is the defining characteristic.

Lesbians face many of the same health problems as all women, but lesbian health care differs in significant ways. Most heterosexual women focus their health care around reproductive issues, pregnancy, birth control or postpartum care. Although these are important for some lesbians, research has shown that lesbians, as a group, seek medical care less frequently than their heterosexual sisters, resulting in delayed diagnosis and treatment (Simkin, 1991; Taravella, 1992). The reasons for the difference in frequency of contact with the health care system are multiple; they include institutionalized homophobia and heterosexism in the health care system, erroneous beliefs held by lesbians that they are immune to certain health problems, and financial barriers to care. In addition, those who do seek care may find that their care is compromised when there is a lack of recognition of their "family" in providing care and support. Many lesbians have responded by seeking "alternative" health care providers, and developing their own clinics and support organizations to provide care and research in lesbian health care needs.

This paper will give an overview of the research that has been conducted on lesbian health care and provider attitudes towards lesbians. A discussion of lesbians and breast cancer will illustrate some of the struggles lesbians may face in finding and using health care in the conventional system. Finally, some suggestions for social work practitioners within the health care system will be discussed.

REVIEW OF THE LITERATURE

The limited research which has focused on lesbian health care has centered around the attitudes of health care providers and the behaviors and experiences of lesbians seeking health care. Stevens (1992) reviewed the literature on lesbian health care from 1970 to 1990 and concluded:

> This review of the empirical literature on lesbians' health care experiences suggests that deeply entrenched prejudicial meanings about lesbian health remain influential in the education of health care providers, the quality of health care they deliver, their comfort in interacting with clients, and the institutional policies under which they work. Knowledgeable, empathic, and fully accessible care cannot coexist with such conditions. The present findings indicate that many lesbians interpret health care interactions as abusive and perceive high-quality, safe health services to be unavailable to them. Such findings are of serious concern and call for immediate radical changes on the part of educators, practitioners, administrators, and policymakers. (p. 114)

Health Care Providers

The attitudes of health care providers towards homosexuality have a major impact on the care that lesbian patients receive. Few studies have been published which assess the attitudes of medical providers, with a published master's thesis being the most frequently cited study in the social work literature (De Crescenzo, 1984), with no study specifically addressing providers' attitudes towards lesbians.

Douglas, Kalman, and Kalman (1985) looked at homophobia in response to the AIDS crisis, surveying physicians and nurses working with AIDS patients. The mean score on the Index of Homophobia (IHP) was 50.84 for physicians and 55.6 for nurses, indicating "low-grade" homophobia. However, the authors state that:

our results indicate that a disturbingly high percentage of the health professionals we studied acknowledge more negative, even overtly hostile, feelings towards homosexuals than they had before the emergence of the AIDS epidemic. (p. 1311)

Nearly 10% of the respondents in this study also agreed with the statement that homosexuals who get AIDS are "getting what they deserve."

Taravella (1992) reported the findings of a 1991 survey of physicians conducted by the University of California at San Francisco. The survey found that 35% of the respondents " 'would feel nervous among a group of homosexuals' and 'believe that homosexuality is a threat to many of our social institutions' " (p. 34).

Finally, a frequently cited study on the attitude of physicians was conducted by Mathews, Booth, Turner, and Kessler (1986), who surveyed members of the San Diego Medical Society. These authors found that 22.9% of 930 respondents scored in the homophobia range on the Heterosexual Attitudes Towards Homosexuality (HATH) Scale. Forty percent of the sample scored in the neutral or ambivalent range, with the remaining 37% being homophilic (having favorable attitudes towards homosexuals). However, of particular interest was the discrepancy between measured attitudes towards homosexuality and respondents' expressed behavior. Thirty percent of the respondents would *not* admit a homosexual applicant to medical school, 40% would discourage homosexual physicians from training in pediatrics or psychiatry, and 40% would cease making referrals to homosexual physicians in these specialties.

While none of these studies differentiates between attitudes towards gay men and lesbians, Mathews et al. (1986) suggest that lesbians are least likely to find accepting attitudes among the specialist they, as women, will most likely need. "The most homophobic specialties, with 30% or more expressing negative attitudes, were in ranked order, orthopedic surgeons, gynecologists, general and family physicians and surgeons (excluding orthopedists)" (p. 109).

Lesbians' Health Care Seeking Behavior

The limited research which has focused on lesbians' health care seeking behavior centers around lesbians' belief that the homophobic and heterosexist attitudes among many providers compromise the care they receive, the research documenting the barriers that lesbians encounter in seeking health care, and the preference of many lesbians for comprehensive health care. The majority of studies are explicit about the methodological problems encountered in studying lesbians, a group which is not easily identifiable and is wary of self-identifying. Convenience and snow-ball sampling have most frequently been used, resulting in an inability to generalize the results. In general, study samples have been composed of predominately white, middle-class women, with above-average incomes and education (Stevens, 1992). Little is known about lesbians outside of this limited sample.

Impact

Stevens and Hall (1988) report that 84% of their sample described a general reluctance to seek health care, and it is well documented that lesbians seek routine care less frequently than their heterosexual sisters. Trippet and Bain (1992) reported that 24.7% of the lesbians in their sample "failed to seek health care" (p. 148), while Bruenting's (1992) study was "consistent with the Smith, Johnson and Guenther (1985) finding that lesbian women are less likely to seek routine gynecological care" (p. 169). Robertson and Schachter (1981) found the average time between Pap smears for heterosexual women was 8 months, and for lesbians, 21 months, using the same clinic.

The most significant risk faced by lesbians in avoiding routine care is "lesbians may not receive early warning of abnormal Papanicolaou smears, endometrial cancer, or breast cancer" (Simkin, 1991, p. 1621). In addition, lesbians may not perceive their risk for cervical and breast cancer to be any different than that of heterosexual women (Trippet & Bain, 1993; Zeidenstein, 1990). Trippet and Bain (1992) reported that the reasons lesbians failed to seek health care were "the lesbians' participation in self-care (as a result of negative experience with health care providers) and the lack of financial resources" (p. 147). The results may be devastating, with lesbians seeking care at later stages of an illness, treatment being more invasive, and with increased risk of death.

Barriers

The literature documents a variety of different barriers to lesbians seeking health care, among them discrimination, including homophobia and heterosexism, lack of resources, and the exclusion of family and friends in their care. Trippet and Bain (1992), in a study of 503 women, 78% who identified themselves as lesbian, discussed five reasons why lesbians fail to seek health care from traditional health care providers:

> The reasons lesbians gave for not seeking health care from traditional sources were that (a) low-cost, natural, or alternative care is not provided; (b) holistic care is not provided; (c) little preventive care and education are provided; (d) communication and respect are lacking; and (e) few women-managed clinics are available. (p. 148)

These authors go on to say that the fear of, or the actual experience of, discrimination "toward lesbians as women and as lesbians" (p. 151) was intrinsic to all five of the reasons lesbians gave for not seeking traditional health care.

Discrimination. Discrimination against lesbians in the health care system is manifested in two distinct ways, homophobia and heterosexism (Simkin, 1993). Blatant homophobia was found in a study by Smith et al. (1985) who studied 1,921 lesbians and 424 bisexual women. They found that only 41.1% of the women had disclosed their sexual orientation to a physician. Of the women who had disclosed their sexual orientation, 58% responded to a question asking them to describe the reaction of the physician to their self-disclosure. While response varied by sexual orientation of the physician, 30% stated that the physicians' responses had been negative. Of these negative responses, 12% were further categorized as "cool," 30% as embarrassment, 25% as inappropriate (e.g., "suggesting referral to a mental health professional, or voyeuristic"), and 22% as overt rejection (Smith et al., 1985, p. 1086). Stevens and Hall (1988) found that 72% of the respondents in their study, who believed they were identifiable to the health provider as a lesbian, reported negative responses from health care providers. "They described being responded to with ostracism, invasive personal questioning, shock, embarrassment, unfriendliness, pity, condescension and fear" (p. 72).

Fear of negative responses keeps many lesbians from disclosing their sexual orientation to their physician. Dardick and Grady (1980) found that 49% of the women in their sample had either assumed their health professional knew they were lesbian or had explicitly told him/her. Smith et al. (1985) found that 46.8% of the lesbians in their sample had told their physician who provided gynecologic care of their sexual orientation. Another 36.4% wanted to tell their physician but believed that "physician awareness of their sexual orientation would hinder the quality of health care" (p. 1086). Fear and concern was greatest among lesbians who sought care from a private physician or student health clinic, while those who disclosed their identity were more likely to receive care at a women's clinic.

A more subtle form of discrimination, *heterosexism*, is also a barrier to lesbians seeking health care, being manifested primarily in attitudes towards sexuality and reproduction.

> I got this survey in the mail, of women professionals. One of the questions was, "What kind of birth control do you use?" I wrote in, "Lesbian sex is the best method of birth control there is." I just wish I could've been there to see the reaction. (Raymond, 1988, p. 18)

Medical history questionnaires and questions asked by providers assume that female clients are heterosexual, focusing on contraception and sexual intercourse (Robertson, 1992; Stevens & Hall, 1988). Planned Parenthood, which provides Pap smears and breast exams to women, mandates that birth-control is a mandatory part of their services (Simkin, 1991). Smith et al. (1985) found that only 9.3% of the lesbians in their study had been questioned about their sexual orientation by the physician, and, as stated by Stevens and Hall (1988, p. 72), "Overwhelmingly, participants found that there was no routine, comfortable way to let health care providers know that heterosexual assumptions were not applicable to them as lesbians." In addition to avoiding irrelevant information, lesbians wanted health information which was pertinent to them.

Financial resources. Not surprisingly, lack of financial resources is an additional barrier for lesbians seeking health care. Dennenberg (1992) discusses this issue, focusing on the economic discrimination women face, and the fact that lesbians do not have access to the resources and privileges married heterosexual women have through their husbands. For example, heterosexual women and their children may gain access to health insurance through their husbands' employment, but "lesbians usually cannot place a lover or a partner's children on their health insurance policy. Furthermore, lesbians may be less able to recruit support and resources from their family of origin, who often reserve such favors for their married children" (Dennenberg, 1992, p. 16). Trippet and Bain (1992) reported that the cost of health care and perceived lack of need were the most frequently cited reasons why lesbians in their study did not have a health care provider.

Exclusion of family and friends. The final barrier for lesbians in seeking health care is the exclusion of friends and family in seeking and receiving care. Stevens (1992) reported a number of studies where some lesbians "only felt safe when accompanied by a partner or friend who could act as a witness or advocate" (p. 111). Simkin (1991) discusses how "lesbians are often denied access to their partners in emergency rooms or intensive care units" (p. 1622). These contexts were also perceived as more dangerous by lesbians due to the reduced opportunity to select their provider (Stevens, 1992), but perhaps also because they felt cut off from friends and family, resulting in feelings of vulnerability and lack of protection.

A number of the studies already mentioned indicate that physicians do not inquire into the sexual orientation of their patients. Lucas (1992) found that the lesbians in her study appeared to have an "ask, but don't tell" philosophy, with 63% wanting the physician to ask about their sexual orientation but only 28% wanting this information included in the chart. Fifty percent were explicit about not wanting it included.

Preferences

Not surprisingly, a number of studies have found that lesbians prefer female providers, and, if possible, lesbian providers (Lucas,

1992; Smith et al., 1985). Moreover, Trippet and Bain (1992, 1993) found that many lesbians,

> being unsatisfied with the current Western medical approaches of medication and surgery, sought alternative health practices that are less invasive and more in tune with the human body and nature. (1992, pp. 148-149)

The majority of the lesbians in their study (77%) did seek care from a physician but did not rely solely on conventional patterns of health care usage. Fifty-seven percent "participated in their health care through active responsible behaviors," being participants rather than recipients of care. Thirty-eight percent "used natural modalities," including herbs and natural remedies (Trippet & Bain, 1993, p. 66).

Lucas (1992), in her study of health care needs as perceived by lesbians, found that they "clearly identified cancer screening and detection and well-woman care as the top-priority health care services they desired" (Lucas, 1992, p. 225). None of the women indicated they were interested in services related to mammography, childbirth, prenatal care, or parenting, among others. Lucas notes the inconsistency between the exclusion of mammography and inclusion of cancer screening as a high priority and states: "Possibly, mammography may be perceived as exploitive medical technology, or the exclusion may be related to the relatively young age of the women" (1992, p. 227).

Buenting (1992) compared the health lifestyles of lesbian and heterosexual women, finding that lesbians had significantly higher mean scores on alternative diet, meditation/relaxation techniques, and use of recreational drugs. Harvey, Carr, and Bernheine (1989) found that lesbians who selected midwives for obstetrical care reported higher levels of support from, and satisfaction with, their provider than those who selected physicians.

In summary, a number of studies have documented that many lesbians respond proactively to the barriers they face in the conventional medical system by renegotiating and redefining health care. Stevens and Hall (1988) summarized the attitudes of lesbians towards health care:

Participants conceptualized health in a wholistic fashion, discussing wellness as a composite of emotional, physical and social elements and envisioning health strengths in lesbians as well as serious health concerns. They focused on independence and self-reliance as the primary components of wellness . . .

The most dominant feature of positive health care experiences reported by these women was the perception that providers accepted the knowledge of their clients' lesbian identity as a matter of routine. This was demonstrated by providers' treating them "like anybody else" and maintaining a calm, supportive demeanor. These lesbian women wanted to feel accepted, respected and welcomed by health care providers. They did not want to be questioned when they chose to have their lesbian partners included as their significant others in health care interactions. (pp. 71-72)

LESBIANS AND BREAST CANCER

The experience of lesbians with breast cancer is emblematic of each of the themes that emerge from this review of the literature: (1) lesbians have specific health care needs that are not currently visible; (2) there are barriers to meeting those needs in the conventional system that are specific to lesbians; and (3) lesbians are proactively engaged in taking charge of their health care both within conventional settings and through the development of alternative health care resources.

Recent studies of the incidence of breast cancer among lesbians underscores the compelling need to identify health care issues specific to lesbians as well as the homophobia-related barriers to identifying these issues. Suzanne Haynes used the National Lesbian Health Care Survey (Bradford & Ryan, 1988) and existing studies designed to determine risk factors associated with breast cancer to calculate lesbians' breast cancer susceptibility. She concluded that lesbians have a one-in-three lifetime risk of developing breast cancer compared to one-in-eight risk for all women in the United States.

This conclusion gave rise to both fear and anger (Rounds, 1993) among lesbians. Reasons for the fear are evident. Anger focused on the possible misinterpretation of Haynes' findings: that being a lesbian is the risk factor. A report in the popular women's press of the study and lesbians' reactions to it underscored the population's double bind. While documenting the need for attention to the problem, " 'It makes it seem as if our lifestyles put us at higher risk,' says Ryan, 'which could make insurance companies red-line lesbians and charge higher insurance rates' " (Rounds, 1993, p. 45). Scrutinizing the research design, Rounds offers a less virulent interpretation, noting "that 70% of the lesbians in the survey had not given birth, a factor that increases the risk of breast cancer by 80%–and puts lesbians in the same risk profile as nuns" (Rounds, 1993, p. 45).

Moreover, while such individual lifestyle factors may increase the risk of lesbians developing breast cancer, more insidious are the stressors lesbians encounter living in a hostile environment (Stevens & Hall, 1988). These are the same stressors which keep many lesbians from seeking care from health professionals, and the same stressors which exist for many lesbians during treatment. Regardless of etiology, diagnosis, and treatment, breast cancer is a devastating experience for any woman, with homophobia and heterosexism exacerbating the devastation for lesbians. These issues are clearly discussed by Bricker-Jenkins (1994) in her moving description of her own journey through breast cancer.

DISCUSSION AND RECOMMENDATIONS

The health care problems of lesbians are similar to those faced by all women, yet the care lesbians receive differs from their heterosexual sisters in significant ways. The differences are directly related to the homophobia and heterosexism that pervade the health care system and its sociocultural context. Social workers throughout the health care system have a responsibility to help eliminate the barriers to adequate and competent health care.

Homophobia and Heterosexism

The first task that social workers face in helping to eliminate these barriers is to evaluate and challenge their own attitudes, beliefs, and behaviors. There is no reason to believe that social workers are any less homophobic than nurses or physicians, and they may be more homophobic than psychiatrists and psychologists (De Crescenzo, 1984). Although, sadly, no one has found a way to eliminate homophobia, numerous studies have shown that personal contact with gay men and lesbians reduces homophobic attitudes. Social workers need to learn about lesbian culture and concerns, in the same way they would educate themselves about the needs of ethnic populations and other cultural groups. There is a large body of lesbian literature available as well as lesbian organizations and events throughout the country. Perhaps the best way to learn is to immerse oneself in the culture, to challenge myths and stereotypes about lesbians. Information about lesbian culture, language, and symbols is critical to good practice with lesbian clients, and in educating other staff within the health care arena.

However, it is also imperative to acknowledge the reality of homophobia and to respect the struggles that lesbians have living in a homophobic society. Asking the lesbian client if she wants information about her sexual orientation included in her chart is important, since confidentiality is an illusion within the health care arena. Not only do most staff within hospitals and clinics have access to the client's chart, but insurance companies may also have legal access.

It is impossible to be raised in the United States and not be heterosexist. Our images and language are bound by the assumptions of heterosexuality. Social workers need to listen to themselves and others in gathering information from clients, and review all written forms that clients are asked to complete. How often is a client asked, "Are you married?" Marriage is a legal as well as social contract which includes a set of assumptions about the relationship which may not be valid with lesbians. A lesbian and her lover may have gone through a commitment ceremony and consider themselves "married," yet their ceremony does not come with any legal sanctions. Such questions as " 'Are you in an intimate relationship with a man or a woman?'; 'Whom do you include in your immediate family?'; 'Do you have a lover or life partner?' " (White & Levinson, 1993, p. 45) will not only provide the social worker with the information about the client's intimate relationships and support systems, but also with information the social worker will need to guarantee the client is legally protected.

Wholistic Health Care

Social work and medicine have some basic philosophical differences about client self-determination within the health care arena (Roberts, 1989). Health care professionals educated within the medical model often focus narrowly on the disease process and believe that their expert knowledge gives them the power to dictate treatment. On the other hand, social workers place the disease within the larger psychosocial context of the person's life, and see the person as a participant in their own care. Lesbians may collide with their medical providers over issues of power, control, and being treated as the recipient of care rather than as a partner in the health process. As a group, lesbians seem to be philosophically congruent with social work, believing in wholistic care and their right to be involved in the process. Social workers need to be available to provide support and advocacy to lesbians when needed.

Family and Friends

Inclusion of the lesbian client's friends and family in the provision of care may also be questioned within the health care arena and social workers will again need to be available to provide support and advocacy. In some instances the social worker may be the "witness or advocate" who provides the lesbian client with the feeling of safety within the health care arena if "a partner or friend" is not available (Stevens, 1992). The social worker may need to help the client obtain a Durable Medical Power of Attorney or other legal documents that establish the right of the client or her designee to be involved in health care decisions (see Ettelbrick in this volume).

Economic Barrier

Lack of access to health care is a problem not only for lesbians, but for 37-40 million individuals in the United States. The National

Association of Social Workers has joined with grassroots and other mainstream organizations to advocate for health care reform, with universal access being of primary concern. Individual social workers need to be equally active at the federal, state and local levels to insure that all Americans have financial access to health care.

However, integral to the debate about health care reform are questions not only of access, but also of coverage, financing, and selection of providers. Controversy about the inclusion of "alternative healers" may have special meaning for lesbians, who often conceptualize health in a wholistic fashion. In addition, depending on methods of financing within the current proposals for health care reform, lesbians may not be economically any better off than they are at present. Social workers need to look at the heterosexist assumptions embedded in the different proposals related to access and financing to ensure that lesbians will have the same advantages as heterosexual individuals and married couples. Finally, given the well documented negative attitudes of many providers towards lesbians, lesbians must maintain the freedom to select providers who are sensitive and supportive (Ryan & Bogard, 1994).

REFERENCES

Bradford, J., & Ryan, C. (1988). *The national lesbian health care survey*. Washington, DC: National Lesbian and Gay Health Foundation.

Bricker-Jenkins, M. (1994). The patriarchy has claimed my right breast. *Social Work in Health Care, 18*, 17-42.

Brownworth, V. A. (1993, March). The other epidemic: Lesbians and breast cancer. *Out*, 60-63.

Buenting, J. A. (1992). Health life-styles of lesbian and heterosexual women. *Health Care for Women International, 13*, 165-171.

Dardick, L., & Grady, K. E. (1980). Openness between gay persons and health professionals. *Annals of Internal Medicine, 93*(Part I), 115-119.

De Crescenzo, T. (1984). Homophobia: A study of the attitudes of mental health professionals toward homosexuality. *Homosexuality and Social Work, 2*(2/3), 115-136.

Dennenberg, R. (1992). Invisible women: Lesbians and health care. *Health/PAC Bulletin*, 14-21.

Douglas, C. J., Kalman, C. M., & Kalman, T. P. (1985). Homophobia among physicians and nurses: An empirical study. *Hospital and Community Psychiatry, 36*(12), 1309-1311.

Harvey, S. M., Carr, C., & Bernheine, S. (1989). Lesbian mothers: Health care experiences. *Journal of Nurse-Midwifery, 34*(3), 115-119.

Lucas, V. A. (1992). An investigation of the health care preferences of the lesbian population. *Health Care for Women International, 13,* 221-228.

Mathews, W. C., Booth, M. W., Turner, J. D., & Kessler, L. (1986). Physicians' attitudes toward homosexuality–survey of a California county medical society. *Western Journal of Medicine, 144*(1), 106-109.

Raymond, C. A. (1988). Lesbians call for greater physician awareness, sensitivity to improve patient care. *Journal of the American Medical Association, 259*(1), 18.

Rennie, S. (1993, May/June). Prevention: Drugs vs. diet. *Ms.,* 38-46.

Roberts, C. S. (1989). Conflicting professional values in social work and medicine. *Health and Social Work, 14*(3), 211-218.

Robertson, M. M. (1992). Lesbians as an invisible minority in the health services arena. *Health Care for Women International, 13,* 155-163.

Robertson, P., & Schachter, J. (1981). Failure to identify venereal disease in a lesbian population. *Sexually Transmitted Diseases, 8*(2), 16-17.

Rounds, K. (1993). Are lesbians a high-risk group for breast cancer? *Ms. Magazine, 3*(6), 44-45.

Ryan, C., & Bogard, R. (1994). *What every lesbian and gay American needs to know about health care reform.* Washington, DC: HRCF Foundation.

Simkin, R. J. (1991). Lesbians face unique health care problems. *Canadian Medical Association Journal, 145*(12), 1620-1623.

Simkin, R. J. (1993). Creating openness and receptiveness with your patients: Overcoming heterosexual assumptions. *Canadian Journal of Ob/Gyn & Women's Health Care, 5*(4), 585-589.

Smith, E. M., Johnson, S. R., & Guenther, S. M. (1985). Health care attitudes and experiences during gynecologic care among lesbians and bisexuals. *American Journal of Public Health, 75*(9), 1085-1087.

Stevens, P. E. (1992). Lesbian health care research: A review of the literature from 1970 to 1990. *Health Care for Women International, 13,* 91-120.

Stevens, P. D., & Hall, J. M. (1988). Stigma, health beliefs and experiences with health care in lesbian women. *Images, 20*(2), 69-73.

Taravella, S. (1992). Healthcare recognizing gay and lesbian needs. *Modern Healthcare,* 33-35.

Trippet, S. E., & Bain, J. (1992). Reasons American lesbians fail to seek traditional health care. *Health Care for Women International, 13,* 145-153.

Trippet, S. E., & Bain, J. (1993). Physical health problems and concerns of lesbians. *Women & Health, 20*(2), 59-70.

White, J., & Levinson, W. (1993). Primary care of lesbian patients. *Journal of General Internal Medicine, 8*(January), 41-47.

Zeidenstein, L. (1990). Gynecological and childbearing needs of lesbians. *Journal of Nurse-Midwifery, 35*(1), 10-18.

Reproductive Issues for Lesbians

Eileen F. Levy

SUMMARY. Lesbian families are often invisible within the national statistics describing family structure and subsequently they may struggle with the question of their own legitimacy. While lesbian families have historically been created through adoption by one parent or children from a previous marriage, it is becoming more common for lesbian couples to create their own families through artificial insemination. However, the homophobia and heterosexism within the health care system deny the legitimacy of this family form. Pregnant lesbians may feel that they have to choose between inclusion of their partners or adequate care. This article reviews many of the issues faced by lesbians as they struggle with the question of becoming mothers, and how social workers can help their lesbian clients address these issues. *[Article copies available from The Haworth Document Delivery Service: 1-800-342-9678.]*

A review of the literature on lesbian health care (Stevens, 1992), and other related studies (Gentry, 1992; Robertson, 1992; Stevens & Hall, 1988) documents the experiences of lesbians in the health care system and the attitudes of health care providers toward their lesbian clients. The health care system is marked by homophobic attitudes

Eileen F. Levy, PhD, is Associate Professor, School of Social Work, San Francisco State University, San Francisco, CA.

Special thanks to D. Jeanette Nichols, RN, for her support, critique, and editorial assistance throughout the writing of this article.

[Haworth co-indexing entry note]: "Reproductive Issues for Lesbians." Levy, Eileen F. Co-published simultaneously in *Journal of Gay & Lesbian Social Services* (The Haworth Press, Inc.) Vol. 5, No. 1, 1996, pp. 49-58; and: *Health Care for Lesbians and Gay Men: Confronting Homophobia and Heterosexism* (ed: K. Jean Peterson) The Haworth Press, Inc., 1996, pp. 49-58; and: *Health Care for Lesbians and Gay Men: Confronting Homophobia and Heterosexism* (ed: K. Jean Peterson) Harrington Park Press, an imprint of The Haworth Press, Inc., 1996, pp. 49-58. Single or multiple copies of this article are available from The Haworth Document Delivery Service [1-800-342-9678, 9:00 a.m. - 5:00 p.m. (EST)].

and behaviors, and the care and treatment of women is based on assumptions of heterosexuality (Robertson, 1992). Heterosexist assumptions create an environment where it is presumed that all women are heterosexual, and where providers believe that they have never treated a lesbian client (Robertson, 1992). The result is both inadequate care for lesbians and lack of acceptance for lesbian parenthood. Because the health care needs of lesbians are different from those of heterosexual women, and because of the invisibility of lesbian clients and prejudice toward them, the situation for lesbians who want to become parents is precarious.

Social workers can, through education, help make health care more responsive to the needs of lesbian families. Advocacy for lesbian-sensitive care for lesbian mothers, and support for lesbians going through the process of pregnancy and childbirth, through support groups and couple counseling, are two ways in which social workers can be helpful to lesbians and counter the heterosexism and homophobia that characterize the health care system.

LESBIAN PARENTS AND THE HEALTH CARE SYSTEM

Health care providers' presumption that all clients are heterosexual places a burden on lesbians either to be open about their lesbianism or to hide it. Making a decision not to come out to health care providers occurs when lesbians do not want to risk receiving inferior care. However, for lesbian couples who wish to become parents, the decision to hide one's sexual orientation can create other problems, such as the invisibility of the co-parent. This disregard for the partners of lesbian mothers and the invisibility of the lesbian family often mean that lesbians' experiences with health care are characterized by alienation. Yet when lesbianism is recognized and sexual orientation acknowledged, lesbian clients feel stigmatized or "marked" and are often ostracized and treated with hostility (Stevens & Hall, 1988). Studies have found providers to be judgmental, nonsupportive and negatively responsive when the sexual identity of lesbians is known (Stevens & Hall, 1988). The lack of confidentiality and the feeling of being on "display" as a potential lesbian parent (Robertson, 1992) creates fear of receiving inferior care for many lesbians.

The importance of coming out to health care providers has been reported in the literature. Lesbians feel the quality of their health care would improve if they felt free to acknowledge their identities as whole persons and felt able to share relevant details of their lives with their health care providers (Stevens, 1992). Most of the respondents in Zeidenstein's (1990) study felt "somewhat comfortable" discussing lesbian parenting options with their ob/gyn health care provider; their comfort depended primarily on the perceived knowledge and empathy of the provider. Lesbians need behavioral or verbal cues from health care providers that convey their openness toward or discomfort with lesbians (Stevens, 1992). If they did not experience the provider as supportive, the women would not discuss their desire or plan to become a parent.

The optimal health care experience described by most lesbians surveyed was one of acceptance of their lesbianism, and being "treated like everyone else." Lesbian-affirmative interactions actively validate the client's lesbian identity by recognizing the strengths and challenges of lesbian relationships (Gentry, 1992). The most dominant feature of positive health care experiences was the perception that providers accepted the knowledge of their client's lesbian identity as a matter of practice (Stevens & Hall, 1988). Lesbians frequently choose alternative health care options to avoid negative interactions with providers. The lack of trust in the health care system means that lesbians seeking motherhood prefer women, and especially, lesbian practitioners, or midwives.

LESBIAN FAMILIES

Social Context

Lesbian families exist outside of the perceived norm of the traditional heterosexual nuclear family. Although there are an estimated 6 million to 14 million children raised by lesbians and gay men in the United States, lesbian mothers are made invisible by statistics that include them with "unmarried" single women. Network talk shows reinforce the perceived abnormality by displaying them as unusual. In actuality, lesbian mothers may have more in common with heterosexual parents than with lesbians who are not parents (Hare, 1994).

Families headed by lesbians frequently struggle with the question, "Are we a family, or are we not?" because of the internalization by many lesbians of societal definitions of family. This confusion is often the result of having no mechanism for recognizing the existence of lesbian co-parent(s). Heterosexist agency forms and policies do not account for the presence of the co-parent.

State laws prevent a child from having more than one mother. Although second-parent adoption is legal in some states, such as California, the overwhelming majority of courts do not recognize the lesbian co-mother as a legitimate parent, and thus, she has no legal parental rights or responsibilities. Even in states where same-sex adoption has occurred, such as California, these rights have only been granted in a few counties. The policy of the state department of social services in California is that same-sex adoptions by lesbians are deemed not acceptable. The social services recommendation must be overruled by a judge, a difficult and costly process.

Because of the often unacknowledged status of the non-biological mother, she experiences a lack of camaraderie and social support from other parents, which can impair the adaptation to the parent role. The second-class status of the lesbian co-parent extends to the health care experience as well. Health care practitioners need to view lesbian families as another functional family system with somewhat different norms and ways of seeing the world. These families continually deal with societal homophobia and heterosexism, and are concerned with their children's ability to cope with homophobia in their daily lives. A study by Hare (1994) revealed that there were no overt homophobic acts against children of lesbian mothers, nor did the children express fear of this happening. Health care providers need to be knowledgeable about the social situations of lesbian families so they can correctly assess the family's wellness.

Issues of Pregnancy and Childbearing

Lesbians considering parenthood are faced with important decisions about conception. They must weigh use of alternative insemination, knowledge of the donor versus an unknown donor, and participation of the donor/father in the child's life; these decisions have both personal and legal ramifications. To choose the best for their children and family, lesbians must have access to information that will help them make informed choices. Lesbians often need access to the health care system for assistance with conception. They frequently encounter health care providers who lack knowledge of lesbian parenting, or whose prejudice toward lesbians precludes them from providing supportive services (Tash & Kenney, 1993).

Many lesbians want to bear children rather than adopt for the same reasons heterosexual couples do: they want to experience pregnancy and childbirth; they are concerned about early infant bonding; they face a lack of adoptive alternatives; and they have a desire to raise a newborn (Harvey, Carr, & Bernheine, 1989). A study of lesbian mothers' health care experiences revealed that 82% of the women surveyed conceived through alternative insemination donor (AID), 65% of them with an unknown donor (Harvey, Carr, & Bernheine, 1989). All these women used the medical system to assist with insemination because they wanted donors who were not gay. Use of gay men as donors has been discouraged because of their high risk for HIV. Gay men donors are also perceived as problematic for potential custody issues. However, lesbians often encounter barriers to insemination in the health care system because of their status as "unmarried" women. In this context, it may be difficult to find a provider for AID services (Kenney & Tash, 1992). Dependency on a physician for AID compromises the personal power and autonomy of lesbians. The cost of AID can be a barrier; the procedure can be very expensive, especially if the woman does not become pregnant within the first few months. However, lesbian-sensitive providers of AID allow the lesbian couple to participate in conception together, if they choose, which can facilitate the bonding process for the co-mother and the couples' sense of family-building.

Pregnancy and Prenatal Care

More lesbian-sensitive prenatal care is needed because many lesbians are becoming parents. Women's feelings about prenatal care are different from their attitudes about the health care system generally. In their study of pregnant lesbians, Harvey, Carr, and Bernheine (1989) found that 100% of the women had chosen to have prenatal care, even though most had not regularly used traditional health care providers. Many women reported negative experiences with the health care system, and were fearful and reluctant to seek medical care, but they viewed prenatal care as extremely important. They perceived prenatal care to be about the health of the baby. Lesbians were generally a highly motivated and extremely conscientious group of mothers during both prenatal and postpartum periods. Because there are so many obstacles and barriers to becoming pregnant, because pregnancy requires conscious choice, because the children are conceived through AID instead of sexual activities, and because most lesbians do not have children, the pregnancy takes on special meaning unique to this community.

Because of the women's prior experiences with health care providers, they placed a high value on finding practitioners who were lesbian-positive. Women who were cared for by midwives reported "extreme satisfaction" with their health care experience (Harvey, Carr, & Bernheine, 1989). Others who used more traditional providers reported feeling comfortable and satisfied with their obstetrical care providers, experiencing support during pregnancy and childbirth. Most women disclosed their sexual orientation to their practitioners, which may have contributed to their level of comfort. An inability to disclose lesbianism can create discomfort in many relationships. Many of the women in this study had middle-class status and thus had access to more of the available resources to seek out health care providers with whom they felt comfortable. In general, poorer women have fewer health care options in many communities. All women may experience decreasing options because of health care restructuring and the growth of managed care, such as access to midwifery.

Heterosexism in medical settings affects childbirth education. It is important for lesbian parents to successfully move through the developmental tasks of pregnancy and childbirth. Childbirth education is generally designed for heterosexuals, and lesbian couples often feel uncomfortable or invisible in these settings. The educator and other participants frequently presume lesbian couples to be friends or sisters, which denies the existence of lesbian families.

The lack of social acceptance of lesbians, and their dependence on social rather than familial networks, raises greater barriers for lesbian couples than heterosexual parents for achieving two critical developmental tasks in the childbearing experience–"safe passage" (women's behaviors aimed at ensuring the birth of a healthy baby), and acceptance of the pregnancy by others (Wismont & Reame, 1989). Lesbians may not be, or have not been, in the milieu of women who are pregnant because so few lesbians have children. They are often excluded from the folklore, wisdom, and experience shared by the community of heterosexual women, where pregnancy and childbirth are a common part of everyday life. The informal support systems of lesbians do not necessarily include mothers. Many heterosexual women do not want to talk about pregnancy and childbirth with lesbians because of their own homophobia, and feelings that lesbians should not be having children. On the other hand, having a child can function as an icebreaker between women and bring out the commonalities among lesbian and heterosexual mothers.

Lesbian women do not always receive family support. The wisdom of one's own mother may not be passed on to lesbians who have been rejected by their families of origin. The lack of informal resources turns women to professionals for advice and knowledge, even though they may be hostile to lesbians. Pregnant lesbians may be more motivated than heterosexual women to seek help from the health care system, outweighing the possible negative reception with the high value they place on health and prenatal care. These women generally receive good care but they do not appreciate the prejudicial attitudes of the health care providers or their lack of knowledge of special issues faced by lesbian families.

IMPLICATIONS FOR PRACTICE

The dilemmas of lesbian families within the health care system are significant. While these women value health and wellness, especially during pregnancy and childbirth, they are the recipients of inadequate care by homophobic providers. Social work practitioners can improve the situation for these lesbian parents in a variety of ways.

With an understanding of the experiences of lesbians in health care settings, social workers can provide support through counseling sessions with the individual or couple. There, women can work through their issues about becoming parents in a heterosexist, homophobic society, and get support for dealing with recurrent hostility and ignorance from health care providers. To help prospective lesbian parents envision potentially difficult situations, these support groups can provide a forum for developing coping strategies through role playing and modeling. Lesbians need to learn to negotiate these institutions in order to receive optimal care. Many support groups for lesbians choosing children already exist within lesbian health care and mental health settings, but there is a need for these resources at hospitals and birthing centers.

In addition to providing support, social workers can serve as patient advocates by educating medical personnel about the reproductive needs of lesbian families. It is evident from the research that lesbians are greatly concerned about the lack of information and ignorance they perceive on the part of the health care providers. Recent books and articles document the experiences of lesbian families; these materials should be available and accessible to health care providers who work with lesbian parents. Social workers in health care settings can provide inservice programs and educate health care workers about the needs of lesbian parents. Lesbians who have had experience with the system can be used as experts and can work with social workers in this educative function. Social workers can play a mediative role in helping lesbians resolve conflicts with medical personnel and in making institutions more responsive to the needs of lesbian parents. They can work for changes in institutional policies and procedures so that definitions of family are inclusive of all families, and ensure that lesbian parents are treated with dignity and respect.

In addition to these interventions, social workers can work toward making policy changes. Social workers need to be involved in the current health care debate, advocating for universal health coverage that includes alternatives to the traditional medical practices for those who want them. Having alternative prenatal health care available is important for the many lesbians who have received inadequate care from the medical system.

Another area of advocacy for social workers is the passage of domestic partner benefits for lesbian families. Presently, pregnant lesbians need to continue their employment in order to maintain their health benefits if they have them, or pay out of pocket for insurance coverage or for services. Unlike heterosexual married couples, most lesbians do not have health coverage through their partner's employer. These heterosexist policies also prevent lesbian mothers from taking leaves of absence or leaving their jobs to devote themselves to full-time parenting if they choose. These same employment policies also affect heterosexual married women, who often lose their jobs or seniority when taking maternity leave, but because lesbian couples experience disparity in insurance coverage, their choices are even more limited.

Social workers can work to change current family policy which disallows same-sex, second parent adoptions. These adoptions need to be made available to all lesbian and gay families who desire them. The adoption system in general is overtly hostile toward lesbian and gay people; the system has virtually shut them out with homophobic policies. Thus, for many couples, pregnancy is the only option available.

CONCLUSION

Social work practitioners need to learn more about lesbians and lesbian parenting, with a focus on health care concerns. Most of the studies on lesbians in the health care system have been done by health care providers, especially nurses. Literature needs to be generated by social workers in order for practices to change and improve. Social workers can increase their knowledge by reading current literature about lesbians, and by attending workshops about lesbians' health care and reproductive needs. Social workers need to be cognizant of community resources for lesbians who want to become parents, and make appropriate referrals to support groups (Kenney & Tash, 1992). Social workers need to examine and change their own homophobic attitudes and heterosexist practices, such as including the lesbian's partner in decision making, maintaining confidentiality for lesbian couples, and ensuring that lesbians who want to parent children are given appropriate assistance and support throughout the process.

REFERENCES

Gentry, S. E. (1992). Caring for lesbians in a homophobic society. *Health Care for Women International, 13,* 173-180.

Hare, J. (1994). Concerns and issues faced by families headed by a lesbian couple. *Families in Society, 35,* 27-35.

Harvey, S. M., Carr, C., & Bernheine, S. (1989). Lesbian mothers' health care experiences. *Journal of Nurse Midwifery, 34*(3), 115-119.

Kenney, J. W., & Tash, D. T. (1992). Lesbian childbearing couples' dilemmas and decisions. *Health Care for Women International, 13,* 209-219.

Robertson, M. M. (1992). Lesbians as an invisible minority in the health services arena. *Health Care for Women International, 13,* 155-163.

Stevens, P. E. (1992). Lesbian health care research: A review of the literature from 1970 to 1990. *Health Care for Women International, 13,* 91-120.

Stevens, P. E., & Hall, J. M. (1988). Stigma, health beliefs and experiences with health care in lesbian women. *Images, 20*(2), 69-73.

Tash, D. T., & Kenney, J. W. (1993). The lesbian childbearing couple: A case report. *Birth, 20*(1), 36-40.

Wismont, J. M., & Reame, N. E. (1989). The lesbian childbearing experience: Assessing developmental tasks. *Image: Journal of Nursing Scholarship, 21*(3), 137-141.

Zeidenstein, L. (1990). Gynecological and childbearing needs of lesbians. *Journal of Nurse Midwifery, 35*(1), 10-18.

Substance Abuse and Dependency
in Gay Men and Lesbians

Sandra C. Anderson

SUMMARY. Research on the incidence, etiology and treatment needs of gay men and lesbians who abuse alcohol and drugs is limited. Recent studies challenge earlier beliefs that the incidence of substance abuse is higher among gay men and lesbians than in the general population. However, a substantial number of this population drink problematically. This article reviews the literature on the etiology of substance abuse among gay men and lesbians, and details important assessment and treatment issues unique to this population. The strengths and limitations of gay-specific treatment programs are discussed. Recommendations are made about how social workers can respond more appropriately to their gay and lesbian clients. *[Article copies available from The Haworth Document Delivery Service: 1-800-342-9678.]*

People who are chemically dependent and those who are gay or lesbian share a history of social oppression and neglect. When gay and lesbian clients have substance abuse problems, heterosexist bias occurs in both their assessment and treatment (Rabin, Keefe, & Burton, 1986). A recent study of treatment providers revealed that they had limited knowledge about how to evaluate and treat gay and

Sandra C. Anderson, PhD, is Professor, School of Social Work, Portland State University, P.O. Box 751, Portland, OR 97207.

[Haworth co-indexing entry note]: "Substance Abuse and Dependency in Gay Men and Lesbians." Anderson, Sandra C. Co-published simultaneously in *Journal of Gay & Lesbian Social Services* (The Haworth Press, Inc.) Vol. 5, No. 1, 1996, pp. 59-76; and: *Health Care for Lesbians and Gay Men: Confronting Homophobia and Heterosexism* (ed: K. Jean Peterson) The Haworth Press, Inc., 1996, pp. 59-76; and: *Health Care for Lesbians and Gay Men: Confronting Homophobia and Heterosexism* (ed: K. Jean Peterson) Harrington Park Press, an imprint of The Haworth Press, Inc., 1996, pp. 59-76. Single or multiple copies of this article are available from The Haworth Document Delivery Service [1-800-342-9678, 9:00 a.m. - 5:00 p.m. (EST)].

lesbian alcoholics and rarely discussed sexual orientation with their clients even though they considered it important. Their training and supervision related to gay and lesbian issues were described as substandard or nonexistent (Hellman, Stanton, Lee, Tytun, & Vachon, 1989). There is homophobia throughout the mental health profession (De Crescenzo, 1984), and bias against research on gay and lesbian issues (Gagnon, Keller, Lawson, Miller, Simon, & Haber, 1982). This has resulted in relatively little sound research on alcoholism in this population, and even less on other drug use (Israelstam & Lambert, 1989). For this reason, most articles discussed in this paper refer to alcohol. The terms "substance abuse," "substance dependency," "chemical dependency," "alcohol abuse," and "alcoholism" are used throughout this paper. There is no consensus in the literature on the precise meanings for each of these terms; therefore, there is a reliance here on the terms used by the author in each article cited.

PREVALENCE OF SUBSTANCE ABUSE AND DEPENDENCY

It is widely held that gay men and lesbians comprise 10% of the population, although a much higher percentage of individuals have had some gay or lesbian experience (Bell & Weinberg, 1978). Estimates of alcoholism among lesbians and gays have been based primarily on three early studies (Fifield, 1975; Lohrenz, Connelly, Coyne, & Spare, 1978; Saghir & Robins, 1973), and have clustered around a prevalence rate of 30%. It should be noted that these studies have serious methodological limitations which include an oversampling of bar patrons who are predominantly white, middle class, and more likely to be heavy drinkers than individuals in the general population (Clark, 1981).

More recent studies have avoided some of these methodological problems and included drugs other than alcohol. Stall and Wiley (1988) studied alcohol and other drug consumption patterns of gay and heterosexual men in San Francisco as part of a larger epidemiological study of AIDS. The gay men, particularly the younger ones, were more likely to be abstainers but also more likely than heterosexual men to be heavy drinkers (19% vs. 11%). Other drug use was infrequent, and occurred mostly among the younger gay men. Gay men used a greater variety of drugs, but differences in frequency of use were relatively minor.

McKirnan and Peterson (1989a) found that gay men and lesbians in Chicago were less likely than the general population to abstain from alcohol (14% vs. 29%), more likely to be moderate drinkers (71% vs. 57%), and likely to be similar in terms of heavy drinking (15% vs. 14%). Seventeen percent of the gay men and 9% of the lesbians were heavy drinkers compared with 21% of men and 7% of women in the general population. Similar trends characterized the use of other drugs. Gay men and lesbians were more likely than the general population to have used marijuana in the previous year (56% vs. 20%), but frequent use was similar at 11% for gays and lesbians and 9% for the general population. Gay men and lesbians were also more likely to use cocaine in the previous year (23% vs. 8.5%) and frequent cocaine use was 2.3% and 0.7%, respectively. Rates of use of other drugs were extremely low. McKirnan and Peterson concluded that, when compared to those in the general population, lesbians were much more similar to gay men in their use of alcohol and other drugs, and both lesbians and gay men showed far less decline in use with age. They did *not* find the very heavy alcohol and other drug use often ascribed to this population.

If patterns of substance use are changing in the gay and lesbian community, it may be due to several factors. There is greater awareness of the transmission of HIV through intravenous drug use as well as the relationship between alcohol and HIV infection. Alcohol impairs the ability of white blood cells to defend against HIV, and some people are more likely to engage in high-risk sexual behaviors when drinking as a result of alcohol's disinhibiting effects (National Institute on Alcohol Abuse and Alcoholism, 1992). Martin, Dean, Barcia, and Hall (1989) have reported declines in alcohol abuse and other drug use in gay men in New York City, and Hastings (1982) has suggested that alcohol use in the lesbian community is declining. This trend may also be due to the women's and gay rights movements, which have encouraged greater openness about lesbian identity and created more opportunities for socialization away from bars.

ETIOLOGY OF SUBSTANCE ABUSE AND DEPENDENCY

Even if substance use is declining in the gay and lesbian communities, a substantial number of these individuals drink problematically. Those who do may be at risk for substance abuse and dependency due to individual psychological factors, social factors, and cultural/political factors. To date, no evidence exists that would suggest biological differences that would inordinately predispose lesbians and gay men to develop a physical dependence on alcohol. If they are equally predisposed, however, the added oppression or unresolved "coming out" issues could produce higher rates of alcoholism among them.

Individual Psychological Factors

Most studies in this category have focused on intrapsychic factors and on establishing a causal link between homosexuality and alcoholism. Small and Leach (1977) reviewed a number of such studies based on psychoanalytic theory and found "no clear evidence that alcoholism is caused by homosexuality" (p. 2077). Israelstam and Lambert (1986) have also called into question early psychodynamic writing linking homosexuality and alcoholism with incomplete psychosexual development.

There has been only one study of the psychological dynamics of lesbian alcohol abusers. Diamond and Wilsnack (1978) conducted intensive interviews with 10 lesbian alcohol abusers and found them to have strong dependency needs, low self-esteem, and a high incidence of depression. Because drinking increased their power-related behaviors, it was suggested that alcohol might be used to reduce sex-role conflict. There have been numerous attempts to connect sex-role conflict with alcoholism, but findings in this area are inconclusive (Anderson, 1980).

Social Factors

It has been noted that gay and lesbian bars are central institutions and that gay and lesbian subcultures may encourage or at least tolerate heavy levels of drinking (Diamond & Wilsnack, 1978). Kus

(1988) and Lewis, Saghir, and Robins (1982), however, found that gay bars do not account for alcohol abuse in gay and lesbian communities. And, as mentioned previously, it appears that norms supporting heavy drinking are changing in these communities.

Cultural/Political Factors

Because the dominant culture in our society is heterosexist, the "coming out" process may involve abusing substances as one way of dealing with the shame of becoming a member of a stigmatized group (Nicoloff & Stiglitz, 1987). Kus (1988) maintains that "it is the internalized homophobia prior to having reached the stage of Acceptance in the coming out process which is the root of alcoholism in gay men" (p. 27). Conflict or ambivalence about one's gay or lesbian identity has been identified by a number of authors as a risk factor for developing chemical dependency (Coleman, 1981/1982; Glaus, 1988; Weathers, 1980).

There is tremendous stress associated with a lifestyle that is not socially accepted. As gay men and lesbians attempt to integrate their private and public lives in a hostile environment, they may turn to chemicals for relief.

McKirnan and Peterson (1989b) have provided the first survey data to test some of these hypotheses. In their study of 3,400 gay males and lesbians, they found that subjects reporting more negative affectivity (i.e., depression, alienation, anxiety, and low self-esteem) were more likely to use alcohol to reduce tension and to use bars as a primary social resource. Stress-related use of alcohol was strongly correlated with alcohol problems in both gay males and lesbians. For both men and women, bar orientation had low but consistent effects on marijuana use, cocaine use, and drug problems. Conflict due to sexual orientation had no significant effects on substance abuse.

It can be concluded that chemical dependency among gay men and lesbians is a multiply determined disorder that is influenced by biological, psychological, social, and cultural/political factors. The relative importance of each factor will vary by the case, making individualized treatment planning imperative.

ASSESSMENT AND TREATMENT ISSUES

It is essential that the therapist develop a respectful and collaborative therapeutic alliance with the substance abusing gay or lesbian client. While it is typical to focus only on the substance abuse early in treatment, some gay and lesbian clients may need to deal initially with issues around their sexual orientation. It is critical to recognize and address shame, guilt, and whether substance abuse is central to the client's problem or concurrent with or secondary to an underlying psychiatric disorder. Common treatment issues include dealing with defense mechanisms, internalized homophobia, and concerns around sexuality.

Defense Mechanisms

The defense mechanisms of denial, rationalization, and projection, ubiquitous in substance abusing clients, may be even more prominent in gay and lesbian clients. This is because these clients frequently deny their sexual orientation as well as their substance abuse and often have legitimate reasons to blame others for their problems (Ratner, 1988). Because denial may be adaptive in dealing with anxiety around homophobia, the social worker must skillfully judge when and how to challenge it (Glaus, 1988). Pasick and White (1991) stress that denial can be challenged collaboratively and respectfully, that it is not necessary to be confrontive and power-oriented. They recommend having conversations with clients in which therapists state their opinions about addiction without insisting that the client agree with them.

Internalized Homophobia

Because gay men and lesbians have been raised primarily by heterosexual parents in a homophobic society, most will learn and internalize homophobia, resulting in self-hatred and sometimes excessive use of alcohol and other drugs. Thus, dealing with internalized homophobia becomes essential to maintaining a clean and sober life (Kus, 1988). Shernoff and Finnegan (1991) note that "growing up gay or lesbian in a family that assumes the heterosexuality of all its members is, by its very nature, a dysfunctional process—unless the family is not homophobic" (p. 128). Children or adolescents with same-sex attractions must develop a "false self" to survive, often resulting in isolation and alienation from their own families.

Sexuality Issues

Shernoff and Finnegan (1991) stress the importance of helping clients differentiate between internalized homophobia and other sources of shame that may have predated the formation of their sexual orientation. While there is no empirical evidence that sexual or physical abuse in childhood results in the development of a gay or lesbian identity, victims of childhood abuse are at higher risk for the development of substance abuse as adults. In a recent study of chemically dependent gay and lesbian clients (Neisen & Sandall, 1990), 70% of women and 42% of men reported a history of sexual abuse. Since there is no significant difference in incidence of child sexual abuse between gays or lesbians and heterosexuals, this incidence of abuse among gay and lesbian substance abusers is more likely to be related to substance abuse than to sexual orientation (Ratner, 1988).

Internalized homophobia may result in sexual behavior in adult gay and lesbian clients that can trigger or exacerbate substance abuse. Some clients cannot approach or engage in sexual activities with others of the same sex if they are sober. And compulsive drug use may be accompanied by compulsive sex. According to Paul, Stall, and Bloomfield (1991), "Sex and alcohol and other drug use may be so strongly linked in gay clients' minds that sex becomes a situation that carries a high risk for relapse" (p. 157).

TREATMENT APPROACHES

Although there is considerable disagreement in the chemical dependency field about the most effective treatment modality, most agree that a primary focus on underlying causation is effective with relatively few of these clients. Modalities currently in use include individual therapy, couples and family therapy, group therapy, and self-help groups. There is little systematic research on the relative effectiveness of each modality with chemically dependent clients.

Individual Therapy

In initial individual contacts with clients, the worker needs to be active and directive. To establish trust and demonstrate that counseling can be helpful, concrete life problems (medical care, housing, unemployment, and similar concerns) may need immediate attention. This should be accompanied by supportive techniques that encourage ventilation about the relationship between life problems and chemical dependency. As mentioned, defenses such as denial, projection, and rationalization must be confronted, although not in a heavy-handed manner. Clients almost always need assistance in structuring leisure time formerly devoted to the use of drugs. Initially, therapy focuses primarily on the drug-using behavior itself. Treatment for those who are suffering with co-existing psychiatric disorders must also address these disorders (Anderson & Henderson, 1985).

When the client's motivation for abstinence is internalized and recovery seems stable, the focus of the work may turn to insight around certain family of origin issues. Issues around loss, shame, guilt, assertiveness, low self-esteem, and over-responsibility need to be addressed in a context of low anxiety so that drug use will not be triggered.

With the increasing interest in viewing problems within a systems perspective, individual treatment appears to be losing favor as a modality. There is growing recognition of the role of the family in the maintenance of chemical dependency and more interest in the use of conjoint and family therapy.

Couples and Family Therapy

The significant others of gay men and lesbian clients may include the family of origin, the extended family of gay and lesbian friends, and a committed partner. Unfortunately, because gay and lesbian clients are often viewed by professionals as primarily single individuals, the family perspective is often not applied to them (Shernoff & Finnegan, 1991).

Adequate treatment of gay men and lesbians who are chemically dependent must take a family perspective that includes both the family of origin and created family systems. Holleran and Novak (1989) note that gays and lesbians who are alcoholic may have problematic relationships with their family of origin whether or not they have told them about their sexual orientation. The difficulty of coming out to parents and siblings is compounded by revealing chemical dependency, often resulting in profound feelings of failure in the parents (Nardi, 1982). At the Pride Institute, a chemical dependency treatment program for gay men and lesbians, family of origin members are helped to recognize that being lesbian or gay does not cause addiction, to come to terms with their own homophobia, and to work through their loss of expectations for their children (Bushway, 1991).

The author of the present paper does not agree with Shernoff and Finnegan's (1991) advice to "provide support to clients for distancing from homophobic families of origin" (p. 134). Collusion with the client's negative stories about family serve to solidify this distance and preclude connections that are so critical to long-term recovery.

Families of creation often play the most important ongoing supportive role in the lives of gay and lesbian clients, and it is very important to understand the dynamics of these families and validate their importance. It must also be recognized that the grief of giving up drugs is often accompanied by that of losing significant others to the AIDS epidemic.

Treatment is greatly enhanced by including the family of creation. As Bushway (1991) notes, therapists need to help clients find a sense of self within healthy connections rather than focus on autonomy, separation, or "codependency." When judged by heterosexual norms, lesbian couples may appear enmeshed. But it must be recognized that this may result from their socialization as women and their need for more validation and support from each other because of prejudice from the larger community (Zacks, Green, & Marrow, 1988).

Pasick and White (1991) note that few clinicians are trained to integrate traditional addiction treatment with family-centered therapy. While addiction treatment typically addresses substance abuse before any other problem and focuses on denial in the chemically dependent client, family systems therapists work toward changing the family instead of the identified client and do not impose their opinions on the family. In interpreting these two models, Pasick and White (1991) propose that:

> The goals of treatment are to support the addicted client while challenging the chemical use, and to support the family's recovery while challenging the under- and overresponsible behavior of its members. The centerpiece is a therapeutic stance founded in part on feminist ideals, one which is collaborative, respectful, non-hierarchical, and appropriately responsible. (p. 89)

Thus, therapists are advised to share their opinions about the existence of chemical dependency, provide education, and recommend treatment, but not to become overresponsible for the client's choices and outcome. Most therapists recommend at least six months of stable abstinence before beginning work on a family and interpersonal relationship (Bepko, 1988).

In working with couples, it is important to assess the adaptive consequences of the substance abuse for the relationship, with the objective of attaining relationship goals without the use of a drug. It is a mistake, however, to assume that shifting the system will eliminate the need for the drug. As noted by Bepko (1989), "The relationship between the addict and the drug needs to be disrupted as well. Systemic change is a necessary, but not sufficient, response to an addiction" (p. 407).

Bepko (1989) conceptualizes three stages of therapy for the addict and his or her family. In the first stage, the focus is primarily on the client and the drug of choice, and the client may be seen alone. In the second phase, the focus is on the client's larger family system and its adjustment to the client's abstinence. In the third phase, the focus is on achieving an interactive balance that will prevent the reemergence of addiction. Bepko notes that the most difficult system to unbalance is one in which both partners are addicted. Beyond abstinence, the major goal of treatment is to reverse ingrained patterns of over- and under-functioning which have served to maintain the addictive behavior. As mentioned previously, long-term maintenance of recovery often requires the repositioning of oneself with the family of origin.

Group Therapy

Because support for changing the pattern of substance abuse is critical to recovery, many professionals favor group treatment (Paul et al., 1991). Yalom (1975) notes, however, that when gay or lesbian group members are in the minority, they may feel unsupported and isolated. Group therapy may be most appropriate when the client is not involved in an ongoing relationship, or is resistive to couples or family therapy. Group treatment can be superior to individual therapy in that group pressure can be used to prevent dropping out and some dependence can be supported by the group (Beaton & Guild, 1976). In groups composed exclusively of lesbian and/or gay clients, there is less likelihood that clients will be able to use their sexual and affectional orientation as an excuse for substance abuse.

Although the primary treatment goal is abstinence in the addicted client, additional goals include decreasing isolation, becoming more aware of and expressing feelings, finding alternatives to the gay and lesbian bar lifestyle, and increasing self-esteem and coping skills. Mongeon and Ziebold (1982) suggest the use of life review, skills inventory, journal-keeping, values clarification, and role-playing to reach these goals. (For a more comprehensive review of group therapy with alcoholic clients, see Anderson (1982)).

Self-Help Groups

Saulnier (1991) points out that lesbians are becoming increasingly disillusioned with both the disease concept and 12-step programs. Twelve-step recovery programs were founded by middle-class, white, heterosexual men. Many groups are homophobic, dominated by heterosexual males, and focused on surrender and powerlessness. Because of this, lesbian clients may benefit more from women-only or lesbian-only self-help groups. Holleran and Novak (1989) found that gay and lesbian clients with a positive Alcoholics Anonymous (AA) affiliation were less likely to be abstinent and those who rejected AA affiliation had greater than expected abstinence.

Bittle (1982) noted that AA has not attracted representative numbers of lesbian and gay clients and reviewed certain characteristics of AA that discourage their participation. One major issue is the insistence by AA members that alcohol is the ultimate leveler and their deemphasis of the uniqueness of the individual. Gay and lesbian alcoholics, on the other hand, *are* unique in sexual and affectional preferences, and "minimization of these differences seems equivalent to dismissing a critical component of their personality" (p. 82). This component is one that the gay or lesbian member may be doubly reluctant to discuss because of AA's general tendency to avoid the topic of sex. Jones, Latham, and Jenner (1980) found that 68% of gay alcoholics in recovery felt that their recovery process would be easier if they could openly discuss their sexuality at general AA meetings (Jones et al. as cited in Paul et al., 1991). Finally, Bittle noted that some lesbians and gay men have difficulty with the concepts of God, a Higher Power, and spirituality since many traditional religions condemn their sexual orientation.

Bepko (1989) points out that many 12-step programs espouse traditional gender roles and reinforce sex-role stereotypes and overresponsible behavior in women. Advising women to "detach" from addictive behaviors is not the same as furthering their differentiation. An alternative program for women is Women for Sobriety (WFS), which focuses on the strength, competence, and uniqueness of women.

Gay AA is the largest special-interest group within AA, with approximately 500 lesbian and gay groups in the United States today. Membership in these groups has been associated with the retention of gay and lesbian friends supportive of recovery (Bloomfield as cited in Paul et al., 1991).

Saulnier (1991) recognizes the general popularity of all of these groups, but questions if any can meet the needs of lesbians, given the groups' focus on personal solutions and denial of political issues. She notes that distaste for the medicalization of women's concerns and for the theme of powerlessness is very prevalent in the writing of lesbians.

TREATMENT SETTINGS

Because few clients are open about their sexual orientation in nongay drug treatment programs, some believe that only the gay community will be able to reach and effectively treat gay and lesbian substance abusers. Ziebold (1978) has given the following rationale for this position: (a) The gay community could become the supportive surrogate family for the gay or lesbian alcoholic without a supportive family structure; (b) If the intervention in the active drug using stage occurs in the gay community, there is a greater chance of reaching the socially isolated gay or lesbian and less chance of exposing his or her orientation; (c) Drug-free reentry into social relationships would be maximized by treatment in a gay setting; (d) A gay treatment agency would provide the role models essential for self-acceptance as a gay or lesbian person. It has been demonstrated that gay and lesbian clients are more willing to attend treatment programs that address gay issues (Colcher, 1981/1982; Driscoll, 1982) and that a majority prefer a gay or lesbian counselor (Morales & Graves as cited in Paul et al., 1991).

In spite of these findings, there is as yet no conclusive proof that gay-specific treatment programs are more effective with gay and lesbian substance abusers. And there are potential problems associated with the development of separate programs. Relatively few large cities have gay and lesbian communities of sufficient size and organization to support separate facilities, and this approach reinforces the isolation and alienation of the gay and lesbian client from the heterosexual environment. With the possibility of referring to a gay-specific agency, heterosexual staff will have less contact with lesbian and gay clients and may be less inclined to examine their own homophobic attitudes. As summarized by Zigrang (1982), the major disadvantage of specialized treatment agencies

> may be that through their separation from the heterosexual majority they may ultimately contribute to the perpetuation of homophobic attitudes that appear to have significantly contributed to gay alcoholism in the first place. (p. 31)

Advocates for integrated treatment point out that programs which treat clients sensitively regardless of their sexual orientation are needed by those concerned about their lesbian or gay identity (Hellman et al., 1989). It may be that the solution is in changing existing agencies, not in developing separate programs. Nicoloff and Stiglitz

(1987) point out that integrated treatment maintains the appropriate primary focus on the addiction and enhances adaptation to the real world after treatment. Vourakis (1983) suggests that both heterosexual and openly lesbian and gay staff be used in programs, since both can be important role models for newly recovering clients.

CONCLUSIONS AND RECOMMENDATIONS

To work effectively with gay and lesbian substance abusers, helping professionals must examine their stereotypes about drug addiction and work through their own homophobia. Homophobia has been found to be positively related to sexist attitudes and inversely related to positive self-concept of both gay and heterosexual social workers (Cummerton, 1982). Morales and Graves (as cited in Paul et al., 1991) studied substance abuse treatment providers and found that 9% scored "homophobic" and 17% scored "marginally homophobic" in attitudes toward homosexuality. Unresolved reactivity about gay men and lesbians can be subtle and very damaging to them and their families (Bushway, 1991). Clearly, gay and lesbian substance abusers continue to receive inappropriate treatment from staff with negative biases (Garnets, Hancock, Cochran, Goodchilds, & Peplau, 1991).

Because it seems unlikely that all cities will be able to develop specialized programs for gay and lesbian substance abusers, it is critical that traditional programs begin a dialogue with their respective gay and lesbian communities. It is imperative that these agencies hire lesbian and gay staff and provide their non-gay staff with opportunities for education and attitudinal change. Suggestions by Underhill and Ostermann (1991) for improving services to lesbians can be expanded to apply to substance abuse treatment for lesbians and gay men: (a) Regular trainings on homophobia and substance abuse should be delivered through both education and process-oriented groups; (b) The Board of Directors, staff, and volunteers of agencies should always include "out" gay men and lesbians. Morales and Graves (as cited in Paul et al., 1991) found that most alcoholism treatment providers reported no gay staff or did not know if there were openly gay staff at their facility; (c) Visible brochures should include resources for lesbians and gay men;

(d) Language on intake forms should be examined for heterosexist bias and forms should include non-threatening questions about sexuality, lovers/partners, and families of origin and creation; (e) Agency non-discrimination policies should include lesbians and gay men; (f) Services to lesbians and gay men need to be relevant to age, race, and ethnicity, and should include the family of creation.

The choice of therapeutic modality for the gay and lesbian substance abuser should be based on individual assessment of psychosocial needs and resources. Couples and family therapy may be the treatment of choice for many of these clients. There is little published data on the special problems of older and minority lesbians and gay men. The prevalence of substance abuse in these subgroups is unknown, but there is no evidence that they are any more adequately or appropriately served than the rest of the lesbian and gay population.

Saulnier (1991) points to the importance of recognizing structural etiological factors and addressing substance abuse in the context of oppression. Underhill and Ostermann (1991) challenge human service professionals to act as advocates for our clients.

> We need to work together to end sexism, racism, and discrimination based on sexual orientation . . . Working to eliminate stereotypes and legal, economic, social, and psychological oppression of all lesbians and gays is essential to building a society where women and men are equal. (p. 75)

REFERENCES

Anderson, S. C. (1980). Patterns of sex-role identification in alcoholic women. *Sex Roles: A Journal of Research, 6*, 231-243.

Anderson, S. C. (1982). Group therapy with alcoholic clients: A review. *Advances in Alcohol & Substance Abuse, 2*(2), 23-40.

Anderson, S. C., & Henderson, D. C. (1985). Working with lesbian alcoholics. *Social Work, 30*(6), 518-525.

Beaton, S., & Guild, N. (1976). Treatment for gay problem drinkers. *Social Casework, 57*(5), 302-308.

Bell, A. P., & Weinberg, M. S. (1978). *Homosexualities: A study of diversity among men and women.* New York: Simon & Schuster.

Bepko, C. (1988). Female legacies: Intergenerational themes and their treatment for women in alcoholic families. In L. Braverman (Ed.), *Women, feminism, and family therapy* (pp. 97-111). New York: The Haworth Press, Inc.

Bepko, C. (1989). Disorders of power: Women and addiction in the family. In M. McGoldrick, C. M. Anderson, & F. Walsh (Eds.), *Women in families* (pp. 406-426). New York: W. W. Norton.

Bittle, W. E. (1982). Alcoholics Anonymous and the gay alcoholic. In T. O. Ziebold & J. E. Mongeon (Eds.), *Alcoholism and homosexuality* (pp. 81-88). New York: The Haworth Press, Inc.

Bushway, D. J. (1991). Chemical dependency treatment for lesbians and their families: The feminist challenge. *Journal of Feminist Family Therapy, 8,* 161-172.

Clark, W. B. (1981). The contemporary tavern. In Y. Israel, F. B. Glaser, H. Kalant, R. E. Popham, W. Schmidt, & R. G. Smart (Eds.), *Research advances and drug problems* (v. 6) (pp. 425-470). New York: Plenum Press.

Colcher, R. W. (1981/1982). Developmental stages of the coming out process. *Journal of Homosexuality, 7,* 43-52.

Coleman, E. (1981/1982). Developmental stages of the coming out process. *Journal of Homosexuality, 7,* 31-43.

Cummerton, J. M. (1982). Homophobia and social work practice with lesbians. In A. Weick & S. T. Vandiver (Eds.), *Women, power and change* (pp. 104-113). Washington, DC: National Association of Social Workers.

De Crescenzo, T. A. (1984). Homophobia: A study of the attitudes of mental health professionals towards homosexuality. *Journal of Social Work & Human Sexuality, 2*(2/3), 115-136.

Diamond, D. L., & Wilsnack, S. C. (1978). Alcohol abuse among lesbians: A descriptive study. *Journal of Homosexuality, 4*(2), 123-142.

Driscoll, R. (1982). A gay-identified alcohol treatment program: A follow-up study. *Journal of Homosexuality, 7*(4), 71-80.

Fifield, R. (1975). *On my way to nowhere: Alienated, isolated, and drunk—An analysis of gay alcohol abuse and an evaluation of alcoholism rehabilitation services for the Los Angeles gay community.* Los Angeles: Gay Community Services Center.

Gagnon, J., Keller, S., Lawson, R., Miller, P., Simon, W., & Haber, J. (1982). Report of the American Sociological Association's task force group on homosexuality. *American Sociologist, 17,* 164-180.

Garnets, L., Hancock, K. A., Cochran, S. D., Goodchilds, J., & Peplau, L. A. (1991). Issues in psychotherapy with lesbian and gay men: A survey of psychologists. *American Psychologist, 46*(9), 964-972.

Glaus, K. O. (1988). Alcoholism, chemical dependency, and the lesbian client. *Women & Therapy, 8*(1/2), 131-144.

Hastings, P. (1982). Alcohol and the lesbian community: Changing patterns of awareness. *Drinking & Drug Practices Surveyor, 18,* 3-7.

Hellman, R. E., Stanton, M., Lee, J., Tytun, A., & Vachon, R. (1989). Treatment of homosexual alcoholics in government-funded agencies: Provider training and attitudes. *Hospital & Community Psychiatry, 40*(11), 1163-1168.

Holleran, P. R., & Novak, A. H. (1989). Support choices and abstinence in gay/ lesbian and heterosexual alcoholics. *Alcoholism Treatment Quarterly, 6*(2), 71-83.

Israelstam, S., & Lambert, S. (1986). Homosexuality and alcohol: Observations and research after the psychoanalytic era. *International Journal of the Addictions, 21*(4/5), 509-537.

Israelstam, S., & Lambert, S. (1989). Homosexuals who indulge in excessive use of alcohol and drugs: Psychosocial factors to be taken into account by community and intervention workers. *Journal of Alcohol & Drug Education, 34*(3), 54-69.

Jones, K. A., Latham, J. D., & Jenner, M. (1980, May). *Social environment within conventional alcoholism treatment agencies as perceived by gay and non-gay recovering alcoholics: A preliminary report.* Paper presented at the National Council on Alcoholism Forum, Seattle, WA.

Kus, R. J. (1988). Alcoholism and non-acceptance of gay self: The critical link. *Journal of Homosexuality, 15*(1/2), 25-41.

Lewis, C. E., Saghir, M. T., & Robins, E. (1982). Drinking patterns in homosexual and heterosexual women. *Journal of Clinical Psychiatry, 43*, 277-279.

Lohrenz, L., Connelly, J., Coyne, L., & Spare, K. (1978). Alcohol problems in several midwestern homosexual communities. *Journal of Studies on Alcohol, 39*(11), 1959-1963.

Martin, J. L., Dean L., Barcia, M., & Hall, W. (1989). The impact of AIDS on a gay community: Changes in sexual behavior, substance use, and mental health. *American Journal of Community Psychology, 17*(3), 269-293.

McKirnan, D. J., & Peterson, P. L. (1989a). Alcohol and drug use among homosexual men and women: Epidemiology and population characteristics. *Addictive Behavior, 14*(5), 454-553.

McKirnan, D. J., & Peterson, P. L. (1989b). Psychosocial and cultural factors in alcohol and drug abuse: An analysis of a homosexual community. *Addictive Behavior, 14*(5), 555-563.

Mongeon, J. E., & Ziebold, T. O. (1982). Preventing alcohol abuse in the gay community: Toward a theory and model. *Journal of Homosexuality, 7*(4), 89-99.

Nardi, P. M. (1982). Alcohol treatment and the non-traditional "family" structures of gays and lesbians. *Journal of Alcohol and Drug Education, 27*(2), 83-89.

National Institute on Alcohol Abuse and Alcoholism. (1992). Alcohol and AIDS. *Alcohol Alert, 15*, PH311. Washington, DC: U.S. Department of Health and Human Services.

Neisen, J. H., & Sandall, H. (1990). Alcohol and other drug abuse in a gay/lesbian population: Related to victimization? *Journal of Psychology & Human Sexuality, 3*(1), 151-168.

Nicoloff, L. K., & Stiglitz, E. A. (1987). Lesbian alcoholism: Etiology, treatment, and recovery. In Boston Lesbian Psychologies Collective (Ed.), *Lesbian Psychologies* (pp. 283-293). Chicago: University of Illinois Press.

Pasick, P., & White, C. (1991). Challenging General Patton: A feminist stance in substance abuse treatment and training. *Journal of Feminist Family Therapy*, *3*, 87-102.

Paul, J. P., Stall, R., & Bloomfield, K. A. (1991). Gay and alcoholic: Epidemiologic and clinical issues. *Alcohol Health & Research World*, *15*(2), 151-160.

Rabin, J., Keefe, K., & Burton, M. (1986). Enhancing services for sexual minority clients: A community mental health approach. *Social Work*, *31*(4), 294-298.

Ratner, E. (1988). A model for the treatment of lesbian and gay alcohol abusers. *Alcoholism Treatment Quarterly*, *5*(1/2), 25-46.

Saghir, M., & Robins, E. (1973). *Male and female homosexuality*. Baltimore: Williams & Wilkins.

Saulnier, C. L. (1991). Lesbian alcoholism: Development of a construct. *Affilia*, *6*, 66-84.

Shernoff, M., & Finnegan, D. (1991). Family treatment with chemically dependent gay men and lesbians. *Journal of Chemical Dependency Treatment*, *4*(1), 121-135.

Small, J., & Leach, B. (1977). Counseling homosexual alcoholics. *Journal of Studies on Alcohol*, *38*, 2077-2086.

Stall, R., & Wiley, J. (1988). A comparison of alcohol and drug use patterns of homosexual and heterosexual men: The San Francisco men's health study. *Drug & Alcohol Dependence*, *22*(1/2), 63-73.

Underhill, B. L., & Ostermann, S. E. (1991). The pain of invisibility: Issues for lesbians. In P. Roth (Ed.), *Alcohol and drugs are women's issues* (pp. 71-77). Metuchen, NJ: Scarecrow Press.

Vourakis, C. (1983). Homosexuality in substance abuse treatment. In G. Bennett, C. Vourakis, & D. S. Wolff (Eds.), *Substance abuse: Pharmacologic, developmental, and clinical perspectives* (pp. 400-419). New York: John Wiley.

Weathers, B. (1980). Alcoholism and the lesbian community. In C. Eddy & J. Fords (Eds.), *Alcoholism in Women* (pp. 142-149). Dubuque, IA: Kendall/Hunt.

Yalom, I. D. (1975). *The theory and practice of group psychotherapy*. New York: Basic Books.

Zacks, E., Green, R. J., & Marrow, J. (1988). Comparing lesbian and heterosexual couples on the circumplex model: An initial investigation. *Family Process*, *27*(4), 471-484.

Ziebold, T. O. (1978). *Alcoholism and the gay community*. Washington, DC: Blade Communications.

Zigrang, T. A. (1982). Who should be doing what about the gay alcoholic? In T. O. Ziebold & J. E. Mongeon (Eds.), *Alcoholism and homosexuality* (pp. 27-35). New York: The Haworth Press, Inc.

Long-Term Care and Hospice:
The Special Needs
of Older Gay Men and Lesbians

Lora Connolly

SUMMARY. The health care needs of older gay men and lesbians are not unique to this population, but the psychosocial impact and legal issues related to declining health are very different for lesbian and gay elders when compared to their heterosexual peers. This article explores the unique issues of older gay men and lesbians, and discusses how social workers and other health care professionals can help protect the integrity of homosexual couples facing declining health and death. Health care providers must be sensitive to societal and familial homophobia which gay and lesbian couples encounter, and be proactive in helping these couples develop the legal protection needed to insure self-determination and the integrity of their relationships. *[Article copies available from The Haworth Document Delivery Service: 1-800-342-9678.]*

While the financing of acute health care coverage has currently captured national attention, the rapid "graying of America" is steadily increasing public concern about the financing and delivery

---

Lora Connolly, MSG, is Communications Coordinator, Department of Health Services, California Partnership for Long Term Care, 714 P Street, Room 616, Sacramento, CA 95814.

[Haworth co-indexing entry note]: "Long-Term Care and Hospice: The Special Needs of Older Gay Men and Lesbians." Connolly, Lora. Co-published simultaneously in *Journal of Gay & Lesbian Social Services* (The Haworth Press, Inc.) Vol. 5, No. 1, 1996, pp. 77-91; and: *Health Care for Lesbians and Gay Men: Confronting Homophobia and Heterosexism* (ed: K. Jean Peterson) The Haworth Press, Inc., 1996, pp. 77-91; and: *Health Care for Lesbians and Gay Men: Confronting Homophobia and Heterosexism* (ed: K. Jean Peterson) Harrington Park Press, an imprint of The Haworth Press, Inc., 1996, pp. 77-91. Single or multiple copies of this article are available from The Haworth Document Delivery Service [1-800-342-9678, 9:00 a.m. - 5:00 p.m. (EST)].

of chronic care services as well.[1] The current public policy dilemma looks much like a see-saw in search of equilibrium: designing a plan that provides enough acute health care benefits for those under age 65 and enough chronic care benefits for the elderly to make the plan attractive to both groups, and yet not make it so expensive that it will not receive the support of industry and taxpayers.

Meanwhile, policy makers and health and social service agencies struggle with a host of other policy issues that impact the day-to-day delivery of chronic care services. Assuring that federally- and state-funded chronic care programs are accessible to all older Americans is one such issue. This struggle has led to an increased sensitivity to the barriers ethnic minorities face in accessing services and the cultural sensitivity needed to make these services more accessible. A parallel sensitivity to the special challenges older gay men and lesbians face in accessing chronic care services is beginning to develop. What those challenges are and what can be done to make services more accessible to older gay men and lesbians is the subject of this article.

GENERAL ISSUES

Background

In 1990, 31 million Americans were aged 65 or older; approximately 12% of the total population. The "65 plus" segment of the general population is expected to grow rapidly for the foreseeable future as the "baby boom" generation ages (National Institute on Aging, 1991). The greatest projected increase will be among the "oldest-old," those aged 85 and over, the group most likely to require long-term care.

Long-term care refers to the interrelated health and social service needs an individual may have due to a sudden or gradual decline of behavioral functioning caused by chronic or persistent physical or cognitive limitation. The needed services range from skilled nursing and occupational/physical therapy to personal care, including assistance in bathing, dressing, walking, and meal preparation. This assistance can be provided in a nursing home, at home, or through community services such as day care centers. Clearly, as the number of elderly over age 85 increases, the treatment, delivery, and financing of chronic care services will take on even greater societal significance.

The hospice movement may be the most tangible example of our cultural shift in valuing quality of life over prolonging life at any cost. Viewed by some in the medical community with some suspicion when first brought to the U.S. in the mid-1970s, hospice as a treatment modality that links the interrelated health and social services needs of the terminally ill has become a part of mainstream medical care in the 1990s. Seen as an alternative to useless and painful treatment in a hospital, hospice care focuses on permitting a terminally ill person to die in a comfortable home-like environment, maximizing the quality of the patient's remaining days, rather than the number of those days (Catalano, 1992).

Some early gerontological studies made broad generalizations about the elderly, using age as a common denominator to explain behavior and outcomes. More recent studies indicate that the elderly are, in fact, a quite diverse sub-population in terms of educational achievement, retirement status, income, health, and social conditions (Butler, 1975; Neugarten, 1979). Ethnic community advocates, drawing on the findings of a growing body of gerontological research on minority aging issues, have pressed for an awareness of the special challenges ethnic minorities encounter in the aging process (Burton & Bengtson, 1982; Torres-Gil & Hyde, 1990). African-Americans comprise 8%, Hispanics 4%, and other ethnic groups 1% of the population aged 65 and over (National Institute on Aging, 1993). These ethnic minorities have been characterized as facing a triple jeopardy: minority status, old age, and poverty. Many of these elderly carry into "their later years a lifetime of social indignities, a history of educational inequalities, lifelong employment and economic inequalities, years of inaccessible medical care and substandard housing" (McNeely & Colen, 1983, p. 119). While the economic circumstances of older ethnic minorities have improved little, the special targeting of federal and state funds for aging ethnic minority groups and an awareness of the need for cultural sensitivity in providing health care and social services has improved somewhat (Hasler, 1990; Torres-Gil & Hyde, 1990; U. S. House of Representatives, 1993).

Elderly gay men and lesbians constitute another minority group, one which is more "invisible," but whose members have also experienced a lifetime of social indignities, employment, economic and housing discrimination, physical and psychological abuse, and often, substandard health care.

OLDER GAY MEN AND LESBIANS

Estimates of how many older gay men and lesbians there are range from 3% to 10% of the elderly population. These estimates could mean there are as many older gay men and lesbians as there are older African-Americans, or as few as there are Native American elders. Fear of disclosure leads many gay men and lesbians to conceal their identity, making accurate estimates of this population almost impossible (Harry, 1992). Older gays and lesbians are invisible because they often seek anonymity to avoid discrimination. But they are also invisible because the dominant heterosexual society more often than not seeks to ignore the existence of any other sexual orientation. Some older gay men and lesbians complain that ageism in the gay and lesbian community also makes them invisible.

Research on the long-term care needs and experiences of older gay men and lesbians is virtually non-existent. Aging certainly brings on new anxieties for older gay men and lesbians as they wonder what will happen to them or their life partners if they are no longer physically able to manage on their own. These concerns are not unfounded. Anecdotally, it is known that many older gay men and lesbians do encounter discrimination when they seek health and long-term care services.

Given the fact that older gay men and lesbians are often a reluctant research group, this paper utilizes a case study to explore the myths that exist about older gay men and lesbians and the unique legal, health care, and social issues they may encounter when needing long-term care or hospice services. Hopefully, this case study will assist health, social service, and legal professionals in becoming more aware of unique needs of their older gay and lesbian clients.

MARY AND CAROL: A CASE STUDY

Mary met Carol while she was living in Southern California. Although she had known for years she was lesbian, Mary postponed her "coming out" until she finished raising her children. After a one year long-distance relationship, Mary relocated to Northern California to live with Carol. Today, Mary, who is in her late-sixties, remembers the ten years they were together as the happiest of her life.

Carol had had lupus for ten years when they met, but when Mary relocated to Northern California Carol was still very active and working full time for the federal government. Mary bought a mobile home which they jointly furnished and landscaped.

After three years together, Carol was diagnosed with a malignant melanoma, and underwent surgery to remove a portion of her carotid gland. Two years later, tests indicated that the cancer had spread and the rest of the gland and surrounding lymph nodes were removed. Carol was told that her condition was most likely terminal and, wanting to get her life in order, she quit her job and applied for disability benefits. With most of Carol's disability income going towards her medical expenses, Mary began supporting Carol financially.

Carol had no real financial assets. Mary had purchased the mobile home and added Carol's name to the title so it would be jointly owned. Although her income declined drastically when she stopped working, Carol continued the premiums on her $50,000 life insurance policy so that Mary would be "taken care of" when Carol died. This was Carol's way of paying Mary back for her years of financial support.

Within a year after her second cancer surgery, Carol began having severe headaches and was finally admitted for removal of a malignant brain mass. The surgery was extremely risky but her only chance for survival. Mary and her daughter, who was very close to Carol, sat through the long surgery together. The surgery went remarkably well and Carol came home three days later. At this point, however, Carol began requiring ongoing care. Nurses came for in-home assistance, senior volunteers drove Carol to her follow-up radiation treatments, and the next-door neighbor came in daily to check on her while Mary was at work sixty miles away. But unable to eat, Carol grew progressively weaker and, one evening, the next-door neighbor told Mary she could hardly rouse Carol that day. Mary called the doctor who admitted Carol to the hospital for intravenous feedings.

While Carol was in the hospital, Mary contacted the hospice program and set up an appointment for the following week to discuss initiating in-home services. But once Carol's strength began to return, she wanted to leave the hospital immediately. Unable to bring Carol home without help, Mary called Carol's family.

Carol had been estranged from her biological family for most of her adult life, in part because they would not accept her as a lesbian. Her family had not seen her during most of her years of illness or even during her hospitalizations. Carol's mother would not agree to come and stay at their home for a day or two while Mary secured hospice services, although she did agree to care for Carol in her own home, some eighty miles away. With no apparent alternatives, Mary agreed to this as a temporary arrangement, and drove Carol to her mother's home.

The next day when Mary called Carol to tell her that the hospice staff would be coming the next week, and that she would be down on the weekend to pick her up, Carol said she was too weak to travel. Mary postponed hospice, waiting for a time when Carol would be strong enough to come home. When Mary would call, Carol's mother would tell her that Carol did not want to talk to her–that Mary "upset" Carol too much, crying after their phone conversations. When she visited, Mary tried to be cordial, but Carol's mother remained cold and unfriendly. On her first visit, Carol's mother asked Mary if Mary was the beneficiary of Carol's life insurance policy. Mary advised her to ask Carol, and when Mary mentioned it to Carol, Carol just dismissed her mother's comments.

Carol had always had her disability checks automatically deposited into her checking account. When Carol became too ill to pay her own bills, Mary wrote them from that account. Two weeks after Carol had gone to her mother's, the checks Mary had written for her bills began bouncing. Mary called the bank to find out why. Even though Mary's name was on the account, the bank was reluctant to give her any information. Finally, they informed her the account had been closed.

During the two months Carol was at her mother's home, her brother and sister made two trips to Mary and Carol's home to collect Carol's belongings. With each visit they took larger items, claiming Carol wanted these things. Mary viewed these trips with some suspicion because Carol was too sick to be wanting the clothes and other items they were taking. To avoid causing friction between herself and Carol's family, Mary did not want to say anything about her suspicions.

Although Carol's mother resisted having hospice because she did not want anyone in her house, she eventually relented. By then Carol required heavy sedation and was frequently not very alert.

Carol's sister phoned Mary about a half hour after Carol died. The family had known Carol was steadily approaching death, but no one had alerted Mary. Carol's sister and mother had been out shopping and her brother was in another room when she died. Carol's sister had called just to see if Mary wanted to come down and view the body. In grief and shock, Mary said "No." She never heard from Carol's family again.

Through a friend, Mary later learned that Carol's biological family had a Catholic funeral and burial, even though Carol had been adamant that she did not want any service at all. Although Mary and Carol had purchased crypts in a cemetery near their home, Carol's family buried her ashes with her father's. Mary remained numb and angry for a long time that Carol's family had not called her when they knew Carol was approaching death. More than a year later, Mary was still devastated that no one was with Carol when she died.

The last time they saw each other, Carol told Mary not to worry, because Mary would be financially taken care of by Carol's life insurance policy. After Carol's death, Mary contacted their insurance agent, who called back with startling news. The beneficiaries of Carol's policy had been changed to Carol's mother and sister the very week Carol had assured Mary she would be taken care of financially. The change was processed through the home office, not through the local agent who would have questioned the change. The agent felt terrible.

Carol had not thought it was necessary to draw up a will because of not having any real financial assets. After hearing about the change in the insurance policy beneficiary, Mary contacted her own attorney. She was told she would have to prove incompetence, which would be difficult since Carol was now deceased.

Mary had counted on the life insurance proceeds to pay off the truck and trailer she and Carol had purchased together. Unable to keep up the payments, Mary was forced to sell them for much less than their appraised value. Since she did not receive the life insurance payment, Mary was forced to postpone her own retirement in order to pay off her and Carol's debts.

After Carol's death, Mary had Carol's name removed from the title of their home, and a few months later she was informed by the county assessor's office that they were coming out to do a tax reappraisal of the home since the title had changed. Mary explained the situation, but had to provide detailed tax records and bank statements proving that Carol had not financially contributed to the mortgage payment. Months later, the office decided not to reappraise the home.

Over a year after Carol's death, Mary was still paying on the cemetery crypts they purchased together. Although Mary made all of the payments, one crypt was legally in Mary's name and the other was in Carol's. Since Mary was not Carol's "next of kin," the cemetery refused to discuss the ownership of the crypt with Mary. If Mary stopped making the payments, she would lose the years of payments she had made. Because the crypt did not have her name on it, and she was not "next of kin," Mary could not even sell it.

DISCUSSION

Just as many early gerontological studies tended to stereotype the elderly, society persists in stereotyping older gay men and lesbians as lonely, isolated from their biological families, and lacking social support. This characterization, however, is far from the norm (Berger & Kelly, 1986; Deevey, 1990), and generalizations about older gay men and lesbians are likely to be as flawed as those about the elderly in general. Many older gays and lesbians have an integral role in their biological family, while others have been ostracized by all or some of their family members.

Many gay men and lesbians acknowledge and accept their sexual orientation in adolescence or early adulthood, although others struggle to conform to society's expectations and only acknowledge their sexual orientation later in life. While some older gays and lesbians find retirement a time of liberation when they can "come out of the closet" without fear of employment repercussions, "the closet" has become so familiar and such a protective device for so many others that "coming out" does not seem desirable, even if considered.

For many of today's older gays and lesbians who "came out" prior to the 1970s, family, religious institutions, law enforcement, and professionals in the medical and psychiatric field were those who stereotyped, rejected, condemned, imprisoned, or institutionalized them due to their sexual orientation. Given such past experience, seeking out and trusting professionals who represent these institutions does not now come easily for these elderly (Connolly, 1992b; Kochman, 1993).

IMPLICATIONS FOR PRACTICE

This case study raises unresolved questions about what might have been done to change the situation in which Mary found herself after Carol's death. In examining the roles of the professionals involved, the discharge planner, the social worker, the hospice team, and the physician, each fulfilled her or his professional responsibilities. But perhaps the most important lesson of this case study is that to prevent this from happening again, the health and social service providers have to go beyond their normal routines and responsibilities.

In spite of her deteriorating health and brain metastasis that had required risky surgery, Carol had not prepared a Durable Power of Attorney for Health Care (DPAHC) to authorize Mary as her decision maker should she become mentally incompetent. Neither felt compelled to do so since Carol's doctors, the hospital staff, and the home care nursing service had all treated Mary as Carol's spouse. Mary could not speak highly enough about Carol's care from these professionals, nor about their respect for her. Legally, however, without a DPAHC designating Mary as her decisionmaker, once Carol became mentally incompetent, her family could have pressed for medical interventions to which neither Carol nor Mary would have agreed. Regardless of age, gay and lesbian couples should be encouraged to designate each other, or another party, as an agent for health care decisions in order to avoid the tragic consequences of situations like the well-known Sharon Kowalski case, where the life partner and the family of a middle-aged lesbian permanently injured in a car accident legally fought for years over who should act as her conservator.

> LESSON 1: Legally, gay and lesbian couples must have a DPAHC in order to protect their right to act in each other's behalf. Someone needed to become an advocate, probing to see if Carol had a DPAHC and explaining its importance for both her and Mary.

Unfortunately, not all gay and lesbian couples have such positive experiences with health care providers as Carol and Mary. In seeking health services, older gay men and lesbians do experience homophobic reactions that range from open hostility to uncomfortable avoidance. When an emergency room doctor refuses to share the prognosis and treatment plan with a gay man or lesbian's life partner (Connolly, 1992a), when nurses and aides avoid the hospital room of a gay or lesbian patient (Pogoncheff, 1979), or when social workers and psychiatric staff quickly conclude that a patient's sexual orientation is the cause of a client's symptoms (Deevey, 1990), prejudice and discrimination are at work.

Unresolved family issues are exacerbated with the stress of a serious illness, and Carol's family acted as might be expected given their lack of acceptance of Carol being a lesbian. However, with gay and lesbian couples, the family of origin retains legal rights if a member becomes incompetent, unless steps have been taken to protect the integrity of the couple. This legal authority extends to personal and financial decision making.

> LESSON 2: Legally, the family of origin has the authority to make personal and financial decisions if a gay man or lesbian

becomes incompetent. Someone needed to help Mary evaluate whether it would be better for Carol to go to her mother's or stay in the hospital another day or two, and warn Mary that Carol might become mentally incompetent after her brain surgery. To protect the couple's financial assets a Will and a General Power of Attorney, which cover financial decisions, need to be executed.

Often health and social service providers look to the families of the patient and his/her spouse to provide social, emotional, and physical support in times of illness. While Mary's family provided some help, the involvement of Carol's family resulted in tragedy for Mary and Carol and the loss of integrity of this couple's relationship. Before Carol's last hospitalization, neighbors were an essential component in Carol and Mary's social support network as Carol became more ill. An older lesbian who lived down the street and had recently lost her partner to cancer gave Mary ongoing moral support. The next-door neighbor took responsibility for looking in on Carol every day.

LESSON 3: Assess the dynamics of family relationships and determine if the families will provide support for the couple or act on their own unresolved homophobic issues. Help the couple explore sources of help within their immediate neighborhood and friendship group, as well as community-based services.

Developing a Practice Sensitive to Older Gays and Lesbians

It is very likely that all health care and social service professionals will be in the position of needing to provide services to older gay men and lesbians. In order for individual providers as well as agencies to become more responsive to the needs of this population, the following suggestions are made:

Learn more about the special issues facing older gay men and lesbians. Educational resources include workbooks on the legal issues for gay and lesbian couples, legal workshops offered through community gay and lesbian groups, gay and lesbian senior organizations, and educational forums at aging-related conferences. The American Society on Aging has a Network on Lesbian and Gay

Aging Issues, and the American Association of Homes for the Aging (AAHA) now includes sessions at their annual conference on gay and lesbian aging issues.

Work through your homophobia and discomfort in discussing sexuality in general. All of us, regardless of our sexual orientation, tend to be reluctant about discussing sexuality in general and have incorporated society's negative attitudes toward homosexuals. One study which focused on mental health professionals found that homophobia was least evident among psychologists, moderately evident among psychiatrists, and most prevalent among social workers (De Crescenzo & McGill, 1978). Working through our own fear and discomfort about sexuality and homosexuality are the first steps in being able to treat older gays and lesbians with the same knowledgeable concern given to other clients and residents.

Become aware of gay and lesbian resources in your community. As this case study conveys, gays and lesbians face many unique circumstances. Become familiar with the network of attorneys, doctors, ministers, therapists, funeral directors, and others who know and serve the gay and lesbian community. These professionals often advertise their services in local gay and lesbian newspapers.

Assess your agency/facility from the perspective of a potential client or resident who may be gay or lesbian. Determine if the questions asked in the initial intake or history presume heterosexual orientation (e.g., "Are you married, widowed or divorced?"). Open-ended questions such as "Do you have a significant other?" create a safer climate for gay and lesbian clients and provide a better sense of the client's social support network. Determine how open the staff of your agency is to diversity and clients who are gay or lesbian. Ask yourself if the partner of an older gay man or lesbian would feel comfortable at a caregiver support group, and if the staff would feel comfortable having him/her there. Also consider whether the partner of a gay or lesbian client is treated with the same respect as a heterosexual spouse, either when visiting the facility or when agency staff visit their home. Depending on your assessment, initiate inservice training programs to educate staff about the needs of gay and lesbian clients, help staff explore their own heterosexist, as well as homophobic attitudes, and revise intake and assessment protocols so they are sensitive to the needs of *all* clients and families.

Grassroots Developments

Although most older people dread the possibility of losing their independence and requiring nursing home or residential care, for many older gay men and lesbians this prospect is even more disturbing. Needing such care might require once again "hiding" who they are or risk becoming vulnerable to discrimination, having a partner or friends ridiculed by staff when they come to visit, and living in an environment that may not even acknowledge, much less respect them.

Aimed at safeguarding the quality of life for older gays and lesbians, special groups are developing in many American cities. The program most frequently being replicated is based on SAGE (Seniors Active in a Gay Environment), a New York City agency established in 1978 to assure that older gay men and lesbians have access to high quality, professional medical and social service assistance. SAGE provides professional social services, social and support programs, professional education, and public education and advocacy. There are now SAGE chapters or affiliated organizations established in one Canadian and eleven American cities, with new chapters in the process of formation. Several women's groups scattered throughout the country are also involved in planning, fundraising, and creating housing and long-term care options specifically for older lesbians.

CONCLUSIONS

Many Americans, and no doubt many health and social service providers, subscribe to the "don't ask, don't tell" approach to homosexuality, believing that what individuals do in the privacy of their own bedroom is their business and they don't need to talk about it. However, this case study illustrates the fallacy of that belief. Had Mary and Carol sought professional advice from a lawyer or social worker, or if the health and social service professionals they encountered during the course of Carol's illness had been more familiar with the problems gays and lesbians encounter, they might have done things differently. If gay and lesbian couples had equal protection under the law, Carol's family would not have been able to close her checking account, change the beneficiary of her life insurance policy, or make decisions for Carol when she became incompetent. Carol would have been buried according to her wishes, in the burial plot she and Mary had selected and bought. Mary would have been with Carol when she died.

Until gay men and lesbians share the same employment, civil, and legal rights as heterosexuals, older gay men and lesbians will be vulnerable to the same injustices Carol and Mary experienced. Seeking those equal rights is a broad challenge to all of us. The more immediate challenge to each of us in the field of health and aging is: "Am I willing to take the extra steps needed to assist gay and lesbian clients in obtaining the care and services they need and avoid reliving this painful story?"

NOTE

1. In this article, long-term care and hospice are often referred to by the more general category of "chronic care." Although hospice and long-term care are discrete types of care, there is certainly overlap between the two terms in the types of assistance the client needs, where care is delivered, and the focus on service providers' custodial and palliative treatment rather than cure.

REFERENCES

Berger, R., & Kelly, J. (1986). Working with homosexuals of the older population. *Social Casework, 67*(4), 203-211.

Burton, L., & Bengtson, V. (1982). Research in elderly minority communities: Problems and potentials. In R. C. Manuel (Ed.), *Minority aging: Sociological and social psychological issues* (pp. 215-222). Westport, CT: Greenwood Press.

Butler, R. (1975). *Why survive? Being old in America.* New York: Harper and Row.

Catalano, D. (1992). The emerging gay and lesbian hospice movement. In R. J. Kus (Ed.), *Keys to caring: Assisting your gay and lesbian clients* (pp. 321-329). Boston: Alyson Publications.

Connolly, L. (1992a, October 15). Learning to protect your civil rights. *The Latest Issue*, p. 10.

Connolly, L. (1992b, December 15). Long-term care for older lesbians and gays. *The Latest Issue*, p. 12.

De Crescenzo, T., & McGill, C. (1978). *Homophobia: A study of the attitudes of mental health professionals toward homosexuality.* Unpublished master's thesis, University of Southern California, San Diego, CA.

Deevey, S. (1990). Older lesbian women: An invisible minority. *Journal of Gerontological Nursing, 16*(5), 35-39.

Harry, J. (1992). *Sampling gays: History and problems.* Paper presented at the 39th annual meeting of the American Society on Aging, Chicago, IL.

Hasler, B. (1990). *Reporting minority participation under Title III of the Older Americans Act.* Washington, DC: American Association of Retired Persons (Series C-29).

Kochman, A. (1993). Old and gay. In K. W. Reyes (Ed.), *Lambda gray* (pp. 93-99). No. Hollywood, CA: Newcastle Publishing.

McNeely, R., & Colen, J. (1983). *Aging in minority groups.* Beverly Hills: Sage Publications.

National Institute on Aging. (1991). *Profiles of America's elderly: Growth of America's elderly in the 1980's.* Washington, DC: U.S. Bureau of the Census.

National Institute on Aging. (1993). *Profiles of America's elderly population.* Washington, DC: U.S. Bureau of the Census (Report #3).

Neugarten. B. (1979). Policy for the 1980's: Age or need entitlement. In National Journal Issues Book, *Aging agenda for the eighties* (pp. 19-32), Washington, DC: Government Research Corporation.

Pogoncheff, E. (1979). The gay patient: What *not* to do. *RN, 42*(4), 46-50.

Torres-Gil, F., & Hyde, J. (1990). The impact of minority status on long-term care policy in California. In P. S. Liebig & W. W. Lammers (Eds.), *California policy choices for long-term care* (pp. 31-52). Los Angeles, CA: University of Southern California, Ethel Percy Andrus Gerontology Center.

U. S. House of Representatives, Committee on Education and Labor (1993). *Compilation of the Older Americans Act of 1965 and the Native Americans Program Act of 1974 as amended through December 31, 1992.* Washington, DC: U. S. Government Printing Office (Serial # 103-E).

Legal Issues in Health Care
for Lesbians and Gay Men

Paula L. Ettelbrick

SUMMARY. The legal system in the United States is based on heterosexist assumptions which place gay men and lesbians in precarious positions when they face ill health or medical crises. This article discusses a number of these heterosexist assumptions and reviews some of the legal documents available to gay men and lesbians as a means to provide legal protection. While these legal documents are critical, they do not ensure that the wishes of gay men and lesbians will be honored if these wishes are challenged by family members. However, executing these legal documents is an important first step in honoring the wishes of gay men and lesbians. Changes in the laws which validate same sex relationships and give lesbian and gay couples the same legal protection and privilege as heterosexual marriage are mandatory. *[Article copies available from The Haworth Document Delivery Service: 1-800-342-9678.]*

A near fatal car accident in 1983 and the subsequent legal battle waged by one woman has done more to instill the need for lesbians and gay men to take legal steps to protect our relationships than any other single event in our history.

Sharon Kowalski was hit head-on by a drunk driver and suffered a severe closed head injury which nearly killed her. In the frantic

Paula L. Ettelbrick, JD, is affiliated with the Legislative Counsel for the Empire State Pride Agenda, 611 Broadway, Room 907 A, New York City, NY 10012.

[Haworth co-indexing entry note]: "Legal Issues in Health Care for Lesbians and Gay Men." Ettelbrick, Paula L. Co-published simultaneously in *Journal of Gay & Lesbian Social Services* (The Haworth Press, Inc.) Vol. 5, No. 1, 1996, pp. 93-109; and: *Health Care for Lesbians and Gay Men: Confronting Homophobia and Heterosexism* (ed: K. Jean Peterson) The Haworth Press, Inc., 1996, pp. 93-109; and: *Health Care for Lesbians and Gay Men: Confronting Homophobia and Heterosexism* (ed: K. Jean Peterson) Harrington Park Press, an imprint of The Haworth Press, Inc., 1996, pp. 93-109. Single or multiple copies of this article are available from The Haworth Document Delivery Service [1-800-342-9678, 9:00 a.m. - 5:00 p.m. (EST)].

93

hours immediately following the accident, Karen Thompson, her partner of four years, tried desperately to get someone at the hospital to talk to her. For hours no one would even tell her whether Sharon was alive, stating that such information could only be given to family members.

Months later, after Karen had spent hours each day waiting for Sharon to regain consciousness and then helping with her rehabilitation, Karen decided that she had to answer Sharon's family's questioning looks about why she was spending so much time with Sharon. In a carefully crafted letter to Sharon's parents, Karen told them that she and Sharon were lesbians who were committed to each other. At this news, the Kowalskis barred Karen from seeing Sharon and eventually moved her to a nursing home where she received none of the rehabilitative care so necessary in those early years. Their action precipitated a legal struggle in the Minneapolis courts. As a result, it would be years before Karen could even see Sharon, help in her health care decision-making, and finally bring her home (Thompson & Andrzejewski, 1988). Karen's legal struggle was the painful effort to reunite her family that had been disrespected and torn apart by Sharon's family, some of the health care providers, and the legal presumption that Sharon's father was her most appropriate decision-maker.

As this account and the many like it illustrate, the law governing health care, property distribution, and personal medical decision-making is both heterosexist and homophobic.

Heterosexism is the unwavering assumption that all people are heterosexual and, for purposes of the laws' treatment, share their closest personal bond with either a married spouse, or if there is no spouse, with their parents or adult children. There is no room in a heterosexist ideology for a life partner, a companion, or a close friend. In fact, it is usually assumed that unmarried adults, regardless of age, are always children under the law. That is, the parents of unmarried adults are generally considered to be the closest legal family members. (If married, a spouse would be the closest legal family member.) Thus, parents will usually retain the right to make decisions for their incapacitated adult unmarried children. An unmarried partner is a legal nonentity.

Lesbians and gay men are most directly affected by heterosexism because they cannot legally marry.[1] Yet, heterosexism affects straight unmarried couples as well, since their relationships also are not recognized by law. While heterosexism can be devastating to gay men and lesbians, many situations are preventable or can be corrected through executing legal documents.

Thousands of legal benefits and protections are denied to lesbian and gay couples, in part because sexual orientation is not covered by federal law (*Rovira v. AT&T*, 1993). Although this lack of legal recognition may result in inconveniences or even serious economic disparity, the feeling of vulnerability and loss of control of our families is most pronounced when faced with illness, dying or death. At these inevitable moments, hospital personnel may limit visitation to only "immediate family," thereby excluding a lesbian or gay partner; a treating physician may feel she is on safer legal ground in following the instructions of a patient's parent regarding continued life support, rather than the unmarried partner; or a judge may appoint a sibling as the guardian of a deceased parent's children over the surviving partner who helped raise them as their second parent.

Of course, homophobic attitudes and heterosexist practices can and do greatly affect the ability of an individual lesbian or gay man to obtain proper health care. However, much of the discussion of legal issues affecting lesbians and gay men in health care consists of the need to preserve and protect our family relationships with our partners, children or, in many instances, close friends who may know more about our wishes than our blood family members.

There are many steps that lesbians and gay men can take to protect themselves in anticipation of illness and death. While many lesbians and gay men are moved to put their legal affairs in order when they are in a long-term relationship or have children, drafting a will or medical power of attorney is advisable for every individual who wishes to make her or his own choices about medical decisions and property distribution rather than have the law decide. The legal steps are important, but equally important in many situations is the role that those who work in health care settings can play as advocates for lesbian and gay patients. Since many decisions are matters of policy, not law (hospital visitation or including partners in consultations), health providers have often been effective advocates in securing equal treatment and respect for lesbian and gay couples. In the Karen Thompson and Sharon Kowalski story outlined at the beginning of this discussion, had a lesbian-sensitive nurse, social worker or physician understood or supported their relationship, a great deal of initial heartache and perhaps legal wrangling may have been avoided.

The best way to illustrate different aspects of the law and the steps lesbians and gay men can take to protect themselves is to provide a context through the stories and life situations we face.

MEDICAL DECISION-MAKING

Marge and Alice, a lesbian couple, have come into my office seeking legal advice. Their visit is prompted by the fact that Alice is scheduled in a few weeks to have major surgery, which will require several weeks of recuperation at home. Though all is expected to go smoothly, the couple figured it is time to put their legal affairs in order just in case something unexpected occurs. Marge and Alice are in their mid-thirties and have been together for nearly eight years. Each has an average income. Marge works for the City of New York and Alice is a freelance photographer. For the past six years they have lived with their two dogs in Alice's rent-controlled apartment in Manhattan. While they do not possess much property, their care and most of their household furnishing were joint purchases. Marge has a modest savings account and a small pension fund through her job. Alice has neither, but does possess a number of family heirlooms and mementos that have been passed down through generations. Though each of their blood families has been outwardly supportive of their relationship, the challenge of who would make medical decisions for them or inherit their property has never presented itself. They are concerned about the legal privilege that their families would have if something were to happen to one of them.

Unlike married spouses or certain blood family members, Marge and Alice's relationship is not legally recognized. Without written documents outlining their wishes, hospital personnel and courts are highly unlikely to defer to their relationship. This fact is made clearest by walking through some of the legal options. While the discussion focuses mostly on Alice because of her imminent surgery, it is just as important for Marge to take action as well to secure her wishes and relationship with Alice.

Durable Medical Power of Attorney

We all want to make our own decisions about health care. Reflecting this value, some state courts have ruled that adults have a legal right to make their own medical decisions. But how are decisions made for us if we are incapacitated and unable to decide? First, a health provider may turn to the patient's family members (parents, adult children, siblings, or other closest blood relative) to determine what the patient might have wanted or what her specific needs might be. This is problematic for lesbians and gay men whose partners are not likely to be consulted, particularly if other family members are available. The better option is to take the initiative before it becomes necessary and designate another person to make medical decisions in the event of incapacity. This can be done through a *durable medical power of attorney,*[2] a written document by which Alice can authorize Marge to make all medical decisions for her should she be unable to do so.[3] These decisions may include dietary requirements, medications, further surgery, a change in physicians or a move to another health care facility. Inherent in the durable medical power of attorney is the right of access to medical records and visitation with the patient. Copies of the durable medical power of attorney should be provided to all health providers so that they are aware from the outset whom they should contact. If possible, a discussion with a treating physician and other family members is recommended so that everyone knows what to expect in an emergency.

But what if Alice is capable of making medical decisions for herself, but is in the intensive care unit? Can Marge visit her if the hospital's policy allows only "immediate family members?" If the treating physician or other health providers know of their relationship or are aware of the fact that a medical power of attorney exists, they can, if they choose, be a patient's best advocate by interpreting the term "immediate" to include a domestic partner. The primary purpose of most visitation policies is to limit the number of people trooping in and out of the ICU. They are not usually meant to make a moral or legal statement about proper family forms. Nonetheless, if the patient's parents and six siblings are insisting on visitation, other action may be required.

Some lawyers would recommend that Marge and Alice execute a *priority for hospital visitation* document which clearly sets forth the people who should be given priority visitation if it is restricted. The legal validity of these documents has not been tested, but often the fact that the patient's wishes are set forth in a formal document may help hospital administrators to defer to the person given priority in the document over other family members. A priority for visitation could be broadened to include nursing homes, substance abuse treatment facilities, and other similar institutions. Again, however, there is no assurance that the document will have any legal effect if challenged.

The necessity of treating a lesbian or gay partner as an immediate family member does not just arise in hospital visitation. Successful drug treatment or mental health therapy may require family counseling. If the center's definition of family is not inclusive of a lesbian or gay partner, the individual's treatment may be incomplete.

Durable Power of Attorney

Aside from the durable medical power of attorney, Alice and Marge should also consider executing a *durable power of attorney* appointing each other to make legally binding decisions for each of them. Again, the term "durable" means that Marge could make such decisions for Alice even if Alice were in a coma or otherwise incapacitated. They have two options. They could grant each other a *general durable power of attorney* which would allow the other to make any and all financial and legally binding decisions. Because it has no limits, it is a very powerful document. Thus, a general durable power of attorney should not be granted lightly. It would enable Alice, for instance, to have access to any of Marge's bank accounts or to make decisions regarding her pension fund. Either could sell the car or enter into binding contracts for the other—no specific consent is required. By the same token, it is an extremely helpful document which allows flexibility for a lesbian and gay family. If Alice goes into a coma and is hospitalized for months, it would allow Marge to sell any of Alice's assets or make other financial decisions in order to pay for her health care.

Another option is to execute a *limited durable power of attorney* which would allow each of them to put parameters on the legal authority they give to each other. For example, Alice could designate that Marge's authority is limited only to selling their car, accessing her personal checking account, and entering into any contracts related to Alice's medical care. By so limiting the power, Marge would not be allowed, for example, to sell Alice's family heirlooms.

Both the general and limited powers of attorney may be drafted so as not to be durable. The document then expires upon the incapacity or death of the person granting it. For instance, Alice could give Marge the legal authority to sign off on decisions or financial arrangements related to her photography business for the period of time that Alice is in the hospital. This would be a limited power of attorney that is legally valid only until Alice is released from the hospital.

Conservatorship/Guardianship

If Alice takes a turn for the worse after her surgery and is completely incapable of taking care of herself or her business, the court may appoint someone to make both personal and financial decisions for her. Depending upon the state, this appointment is called a conservatorship or guardianship. Since Alice runs her own freelance business, this might be particularly important for her to consider. Though the court appointment would not occur unless or until she is incapacitated, Alice may sign a document nominating Marge to be her conservator or guardian. Marge could then petition the court to be appointed as Alice's conservator by proving that Alice is legally incapacitated from making decisions for herself and that Marge is the best person to oversee Alice's personal and business concerns. The appointment would allow Marge to take care of routine business matters such as paying business-related bills out of Alice's business accounts, issuing paychecks to employees, or entering into contracts. She could also handle extraordinary matters such as liquidating Alice's business. With the court's approval, Marge's duties could extend beyond Alice's business to her personal affairs, like selling any possessions Alice might have in order to pay for medical expenses and making sure that her physical needs for food, housing and health care are provided for.

In the absence of a nomination of conservatorship, courts would more likely appoint a blood family member over a lesbian or gay lover, especially if there were a dispute between the love and blood relative. Although Alice's nomination of Marge does not absolutely ensure that the court will appoint Marge if Alice's family challenges the appointment, it does put Marge in a much stronger position than she would be without the nomination.

Conservatorships are not always the most desirable method for caring for someone. Marge would need court approval for most decisions she would make, and all decisions would become part of a public record through the court. Also, the legal fees and other expenses of a conservatorship make it costly. Most of the necessary decisions can be provided through other arrangements like the various powers of attorney.

Living Will

With the advent of medical technology that can mechanically prolong a patient's life, most states have passed laws allowing an individual to direct her or his physician in advance to either not apply or to remove artificial life-support systems if her or his medical condition is terminal and irreversible. The documents, called either *living wills* or *advance directives*, are written statements addressed directly to any treating physician stating the patient's wishes. Life support is never removed unless it is proven that the patient would have wanted such drastic action taken. A living will gives one the opportunity to make that decision explicit. While most physicians will consult with family members and, hopefully, lesbian and gay partners before removing life support systems, the living will requires the physician to follow the patient's directive, which cannot be overruled absent formal legal proceedings. In contrast to the power of attorney, the living will addresses *only* the decision regarding life-sustaining treatments or "do not resuscitate" orders.

To be valid, the living will must conform precisely to the procedure outlined in the state law. The patient's intent must be very explicitly stated. It is always advisable to discuss the matter with the treating physician and to provide her or him with a copy of the living will to be included in the medical records. It is also wise to provide an original copy to a partner or trusted friend or family member.

In the absence of a living will, some state laws provide that family members or others close to the patient be granted the legal authority to act as surrogate decision-maker in deciding whether to remove life support. That person must be close enough to have reason to know what the patient might have wanted regarding life support. These laws give family members priority, directing that physicians should first consult the patient's spouse; if no spouse, then a parent; if no parent, then an adult child, etc. In New York, the statute also includes a close friend, though that person is listed as the last priority. It may be argued, however, that if Marge holds Alice's durable medical power of attorney she should be the priority surrogate decision-maker.

Marge and Alice should be prompted to seriously discuss their views on this matter and to let each other know their wishes. Certainly, the only downside to not drafting a living will is that most medical providers will assume that life support is desired. Though this assumption errs on the ethical side of keeping the person alive, it may prolong the emotional turmoil for family members indefinitely, especially if the patient is in a persistent vegetative state. However, if Alice felt strongly that life support should not be resorted to, Marge would have to incur the agony and legal expense of a court proceeding proving that Alice did not want life support and seeking an order to disconnect her from such support in the absence of a living will. It is much easier all the way around to simply execute the appropriate documents, assuming that is her wish.

One caveat should be noted. While many courts and legislatures have decided that patients have a legal right to make their own medical decisions, including discontinuation of life support, this issue raises personal concerns for all involved. Some hospitals, particularly religious hospitals, may decide that discontinuing life support violates religious and ethical principles. As a constitutional principle, they may be within their First Amendment right to freedom of religion to refuse to discontinue life support. Thus, Alice should check the hospital's policy before surgery. In the event that the hospital has such a policy, she should be aware of two options. She may go to another hospital, a decision complicated by the possibility that her surgeon may not have privileges to perform surgery at other hospitals. Or, having given Marge her durable medical power of attorney as discussed earlier, Marge can use the power of attorney to decide to move Alice to another hospital that will honor the living will.

RELATED LEGAL ISSUES

Domestic Partnership

Although many of the legal steps discussed are available throughout the country, other procedures that are less well developed in law may provide additional protection for lesbians and gay men. One such area is domestic partnership: an unmarried, non-sanguine relationship recognized by an employer, government body, or some other entity for purposes of providing certain benefits conferring limited legal recognition of the relationship. At its inception, domestic partnership was promoted more as an equality issue rather than a relationship recognition issue. Most employment benefits policies, for example, provide health insurance, family sick leave, bereavement leave, tuition reimbursement, and a host of other economic benefits only to the legal spouses and children of its employees. Employees who are unmarried, but sharing their lives with committed life partners and children, are denied these economic benefits. They receive fewer benefits from their employer than their married co-workers and, as a result, are paid less. Not only are they paid less, but they must often incur the out-of-pocket cost of health insurance for their partners or take vacation time as a substitute for bereavement leave or family sick leave, which is readily available for married employees.[4] Lesbian and gay couples in particular are put in an impossible position because they are not allowed to marry in order to receive benefits.

Since the mid-1980s, the lesbian and gay community, in particular, has successfully advocated for domestic partner benefits in an array of employment and civic arenas. While the vast majority of employers still provide benefits only to married employees, a growing number of private employers, cities, and universities provide benefits on an equal basis to married and unmarried employees alike. Further, while most employers have not made the economic leap to provide health insurance benefits, many have revised their personnel policies with regard to issues like paid bereavement leave and family sick leave.

Returning briefly to Marge and Alice, note that Marge works for the City of New York, which happens to provide the full range of benefits for domestic partners of city workers. Since Alice is self-employed (thus probably either uninsured or underinsured), they have the option to register with the city clerk's office as domestic partners, which would be the first step towards allowing Marge to put Alice on her employer health insurance plan. In addition to health insurance, Marge is also entitled to a set number of days of paid family sick leave to care for Alice during her recuperation. Should Alice die, Marge would also receive paid bereavement leave.

Since they live in a city that recognizes domestic partner relationships, upon registering, Marge and Alice would be entitled to other benefits even if Marge were not employed by the City. Of relevance here is the guarantee that Marge would have hospital visitation privileges on a par with other family members if Alice were in any city-run hospital.

Will and Testament

James and Carlos are a gay couple with two children, both of whom are Carlos' biological children from a prior marriage. The children have lived with Carlos since his wife (their mother) died eight years ago. James moved into their home, which Carlos owns, and joined their family five years ago. James contributes equally to the household expenses and is as devoted to the children and their well-being as Carlos. For their part, the children adore him and have come to consider James their second father. Carlos has just been diagnosed with AIDS.

He and James are concerned about what will become of the children, their home and their possessions should Carlos die.

James and Carlos should consider executing all of the documents already recommended for Marge and Alice to assist them in dealing with inevitable hospitalization and medical decision-making. Also, they should each execute a *last will and testament*. A will is the legal declaration by an individual as to how his property should be distributed and his estate administered. By definition, a will becomes effective only upon death. It may be amended or revoked at any time (and as many times as one wishes) prior to death.

Every adult is legally capable of executing a will so long as she or he is mentally competent to do so. Deathbed wills should be avoided because they may raise the issue of the mental competence of the individual executing it. Many a will has been challenged by disgruntled family members on the grounds that the deceased individual lacked the required legal capacity to execute or amend the will in those final days before death. If the will is executed in the hospital, hospice or nursing home, health providers and others attending to the needs of the individual should carefully document his mental capacity in the event that the will is challenged.

If the will is overturned because the testator (the person who executes the will) lacked requisite mental capacity, the estate will be treated as if he or she never had a will. That is, the law will presume that the testator intended his/her property to go to any surviving spouse, children, parents, or other statutorily determined blood family members, and will require distribution accordingly. The law does not recognize the right of a surviving domestic partner to inherit the property of a deceased partner unless such a provision is made in the will.

A will is an essential vehicle for Carlos and James to make a range of decisions. In their respective wills, they can each state that they want some or all of their property to go to each other. Carlos, who owns the home in which they live, may especially wish to leave the house to James so that he and the children will have a secure place to live. Carlos may also wish to make a special financial provision for the children by using his will to set up a trust for the children and designating that a certain portion of his assets go into the trust. Since the children are not adults, it would not be wise to leave the money to them directly to use in whatever way they might choose. A trust would assure that the money is used for the exclusive well-being of the children, and the trustee is accountable to the court for the finances of the trust. James also could establish a trust for the children even though they are not his biological children. Although most states do not allow an individual to disinherit a spouse, there are no other limitations as to whom property may be left through a will.

A will allows for decision-making beyond property distribution and, thus, is an important document to consider even for those who do not own much property. For instance, in his will, Carlos may nominate James as the guardian for his children. While a nomination of guardianship in the will is the most traditionally accepted means for letting the judge know of the parent's wishes after death, the court is not bound by the nomination. If other relatives challenge the nomination on the grounds that it is not in the children's best interests to live with a gay man who is not their legal father, the court would not necessarily be required to appoint James as the guardian, a situation which would not give Carlos and James much comfort.

The AIDS crisis has spurred many legal reforms, one of which is legislation in a handful of states allowing for the appointment of a *stand-by guardian*. Primarily because of the experiences of women with HIV who wanted some assurance about what would become of their children after they died, legislation was passed in New York, Florida and perhaps a few other states to allow an ill parent to designate a guardian to be appointed after the parent's death. Unlike the nomination of a guardian in a will, the stand-by guardianship procedure assures the appointment of the designated person, providing a more modern and humane solution for ill parents. If they live in a state with a stand-by guardianship law, Carlos would be wiser to follow the provision of that statute to establish a legal guardian for his child. Should he die and James becomes the children's guardian, he should consider filing a petition to adopt them as soon as possible.

Another legal step that they should inquire about is that of a *second-parent adoption*, whereby James, with Carlos' consent, would petition the court to adopt Carlos' children as their second parent. The legal effect of a second-parent adoption is that both Carlos and James would be fully legal parents of the children. This is still a very novel proceeding and should be carefully investigated before proceeding. Vermont and Massachusetts are thus far the only states that allow second-parent adoptions. In other states, individual judges have been willing to grant them, mostly in the larger cities like Minneapolis, San Antonio, Seattle, San Francisco, New York (Manhattan only), and Chicago. With a second-parent adoption, the children would be legally James' children as well as Carlos', and would more likely stay in his custody should Carlos die.[5] James would be liable for the children's support and could make health care decisions for them.

Carlos and James may also provide for funeral and burial arrangements in their wills, a particularly important provision for a person whose individual wishes may run contrary to those of his/her blood family. For instance, if Carlos does not want the Catholic funeral which he knows his parents would arrange, but would prefer cremation and a memorial service, he must make his wishes known in his will. He should set forth his wishes, any arrangements he has already made and paid for, and the disposition, if any, of anatomical parts. Because a will takes some time to be formally probated, a process that will not be completed until long after death, Carlos and James should be sure that friends and family members are told ahead of time of their wishes. Paying for the arrangements before death is a good sign of intent. Without a will or any other tangible sign of intentions regarding burial or services, most states allow the "next of kin" (usually, spouse or blood family) to take possession of the body.

A will also allows Carlos and James to appoint an executor whose job it is to oversee and enforce all provisions of the will. This responsibility would include, for instance, making sure that burial or guardianship provisions are adhered to. It is a position of great trust. Carlos and James would most likely want to appoint each other to be executor and to name other close friends as alternatives should they die at the same time or are otherwise unable to function as an executor because of their own illness or incapacity.

Joint Property

After death, a will is submitted to the court for probate. Since probating a will takes time and costs money that could be better used by the surviving partner to pay expenses or debts, it is wise to consider owning property jointly with the person who would inherit it anyway. Thus, Carlos should consider changing the deed to his house from sole ownership to "joint ownership with a right of survivorship" with James. This way, if Carlos dies, James will automatically own the home. In addition, this form of ownership removes the home from the will, which means it is beyond the reach of Carlos' family members should they challenge the will.

Bank accounts and many other financial funds may also be owned jointly with rights of survivorship, so that upon Carlos' death, money in the account would automatically belong to James and vice versa. James would then have immediate access to all of the funds to continue paying the mortgage, hospital bills, or to provide for the children. This course is advisable because it ensures that a surviving partner has enough money to hold him/her over until life insurance proceeds are paid and/or the will is probated. One should always be aware of a potential pitfall of joint accounts: either party to a joint account may withdraw all of the funds at any time.

Lesbians and gay men typically fear that blood family members will be able to successfully challenge their wills, particularly if they leave all or most of their property to their lover, to lesbian or gay friends or organizations. If the will is properly drafted and executed, the person is of sound mind and there was no fraud or undue influence by one of the beneficiaries of the will, it is highly unlikely that a family member will succeed in overturning the will. The sexual orientation either of the person drafting the will or the beneficiary is not a basis of overturning a will. (Of course, there is nothing that can actually prevent a family member from filing a challenge to the will, no matter how frivolous the grounds.) The best policy for James and Carlos, as well as Marge and Alice, would be to let their families know of the contents of their respective wills ahead of time so that they can personally explain their wishes and let family members get used to them in order to avert any trouble after death.

CONCLUSION

Only full legal and societal respect for lesbian and gay families will assure that their family lives will proceed without additional trauma at a time of illness or tragedy. This article is only able to touch briefly on a few of the issues that might arise for lesbians and gay men when they deal with health care systems. Two points are most important. First, taking some action to draft legal documents or pursue legal proceedings is critical to gay men and lesbians who want to have their medical and personal wishes, as well as the integrity of their relationships, honored. Second, as important as these documents are, there is no substitute for having supportive advocates within the health care setting to see that health care providers treat lesbian and gay patients with the same respect expected for every patient.

NOTES

1. Recently, though, the Hawaii Supreme Court opened the first legal door to the possibility of lesbian and gay marriages. In *Baehr v. Lewin* (1993), the court ruled that the laws allowing only heterosexual couples to marry may be unconstitutionally discriminatory unless the state can show a compelling reason for denying the right of marriage to lesbian and gay couples.

2. Many states have passed legislation explicitly allowing for medical powers of attorney and setting forth their requirements. In other states, the validity of these documents is assumed under the general presumption that each person has a right to make her own decisions. An extension of that right is the right to appoint another person of one's own choice to make those decisions in the event of incapacity.

3. Most powers of attorney expire upon the death or incapacity of the person giving the power. The term *durable* indicates that it can be used even if the patient is physically or mentally incapable of making a decision for herself. Medical powers of attorney should always state that they are durable, since their primary purpose is to allow another person to make decisions for someone incapable of doing so. If Alice *could* make her own medical decision, she would not need the durable medical power of attorney. By contrast, a *power of attorney* that is not designated to apply to medical decisions is used to authorize an agent to make decisions in other contexts, usually financial transactions.

4. For more complete discussion of domestic partnership benefits and advocacy, the following organizations have helpful publications: Lambda Legal Defense and Education Fund, 666 Broadway, NY, NY 10012; National Gay and Lesbian Task Force, 2320 17th Street, NW, Washington, DC 20009; and National Center for Lesbian Rights, 870 Market Street, Suite 570, San Francisco, CA 94102.

5. Unfortunately, we must always keep in mind that nothing is certain for lesbian and gay parents. If Carlos' blood family wanted to challenge James' custody of the children on the grounds that the fact that he is gay makes him unfit to be a parent, there are still many judges who would remove the children from his custody. If he is their adoptive father, it is much more difficult, though not impossible, to take the children away.

REFERENCES

Baehr v. Lewin, 852P.2d.44 (Hawaii Sup. Ct. 1993).
Rovira v. AT&T, 760F. Supp. 376 (1993).
Thompson, K. & Andrzejewski, J. (1988). *Why can't Sharon Kowalski come home?* San Francisco: Spinsters/Aunt Lute.

Index

Notes: Page numbers followed by "n" indicates end-of-chapter Notes.

Page numbers preceded by *mentioned* indicates intermittent discussion of the subject on all inclusive pages.

Adolescents. *See* Youth
Adoption of children 52,53,57,
    105-106
African-Americans 79,80
Age
    of acknowledgment/acceptance of
       homosexual orientation
       4,85
    of first same-sex activity 4
    as substance abuse factor 60-61
Aged persons. *See* Chronic health
       care; Older gay men and
       lesbians
Agencies. *See* Health care agencies
AIDS/HIV
    grief of survivors 67
    homosexuality issues
       subordinated by attention to
       11
    impact on attitudes of health
       professionals toward
       homosexuality 21,35-36
    and legal reforms for child
       guardianship 105
    service organizations and
       activism 21,22,30,31
    transmission/infection
       adolescents' risks 8
       gay men as alternative
        insemination donors 53

ignorance and misconceptions
    of health professionals
    21-22,25,26
substance abuse related to 26,
    61
women undiagnosed by
    physicians 26
AIDS/HIV, persons with: health
    providers' attitudes and
    treatment practices toward
benign neglect 21,23-24
compassionate practices 28-29
confidentiality and violations
    27-28,29
irrational fears 21,23,25,26,27
refusal of treatment 21,22,26
toward substance abusers 26
toward women 26
Alcoholics Anonymous (AA) 69-70
    Gay AA 70
Alcoholism; alcohol use 5,8;
    mentioned 60-70. *See also*
    Substance abuse
American Academy of Pediatrics 2
American Association of Homes for
    the Aging 88
American Medical Association 2
American Society on Aging 87-88

    111

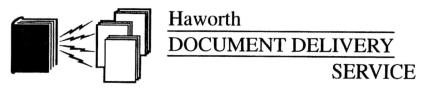

Haworth
DOCUMENT DELIVERY
SERVICE

This valuable service provides a single-article order form for any article from a Haworth journal.

- *Time Saving:* No running around from library to library to find a specific article.
- *Cost Effective:* All costs are kept down to a minimum.
- *Fast Delivery:* Choose from several options, including same-day FAX.
- *No Copyright Hassles:* You will be supplied by the original publisher.
- *Easy Payment:* Choose from several easy payment methods.

Open Accounts Welcome for . . .
- Library Interlibrary Loan Departments
- Library Network/Consortia Wishing to Provide Single-Article Services
- Indexing/Abstracting Services with Single Article Provision Services
- Document Provision Brokers and Freelance Information Service Providers

---

MAIL or *FAX* THIS ENTIRE ORDER FORM TO:

Haworth Document Delivery Service
The Haworth Press, Inc.
10 Alice Street
Binghamton, NY 13904-1580

or FAX: 1-800-895-0582
or CALL: 1-800-342-9678
9am-5pm EST

PLEASE SEND ME PHOTOCOPIES OF THE FOLLOWING SINGLE ARTICLES:

1) Journal Title: _____
   Vol/Issue/Year:_____Starting & Ending Pages:_____
Article Title:_____

2) Journal Title: _____
   Vol/Issue/Year:_____Starting & Ending Pages:_____
Article Title:_____

3) Journal Title: _____
   Vol/Issue/Year:_____Starting & Ending Pages:_____
Article Title:_____

4) Journal Title: _____
   Vol/Issue/Year:_____Starting & Ending Pages:_____
Article Title:_____

(See other side for Costs and Payment Information)

COSTS: Please figure your cost to order quality copies of an article.

1. Set-up charge per article: $8.00

            ($8.00 × number of separate articles) _____

2. Photocopying charge for each article:

            1-10 pages: $1.00 _____

            11-19 pages: $3.00 _____

            20-29 pages: $5.00 _____

            30+ pages: $2.00/10 pages _____

3. Flexicover (optional): $2.00/article _____

4. Postage & Handling: US: $1.00 for the first article/

            $.50 each additional article _____

            Federal Express: $25.00 _____

            Outside US: $2.00 for first article/

            $.50 each additional article _____

5. Same-day FAX service: $.35 per page _____

                          GRAND TOTAL: _____

METHOD OF PAYMENT: (please check one)

❏ Check enclosed   ❏ Please ship and bill. PO # _____

        (sorry we can ship and bill to bookstores only! All others must pre-pay)

❏ Charge to my credit card: ❏ Visa; ❏ MasterCard; ❏ Discover;

        ❏ American Express;

Account Number:_____ Expiration date:_____

Signature: ✗_____

Name: _____ Institution: _____

Address: _____

_____

City: _____ State:_____ Zip:_____

Phone Number: _____ FAX Number: _____

MAIL or *FAX* THIS ENTIRE ORDER FORM TO:

Haworth Document Delivery Service	**or FAX:** 1-800-895-0582
The Haworth Press, Inc.	**or CALL:** 1-800-342-9678
10 Alice Street	9am-5pm EST)
Binghamton, NY 13904-1580	